Non-Operative Treatment of the Lumbar Spine

Grant Cooper

Non-Operative Treatment of the Lumbar Spine

Springer

Grant Cooper
Princeton Spine & Joint Center
Princeton, NJ, USA

ISBN 978-3-319-21442-9 ISBN 978-3-319-21443-6 (eBook)
DOI 10.1007/978-3-319-21443-6

Library of Congress Control Number: 2015946605

Springer Cham Heidelberg New York Dordrecht London

Printed on acid-free paper

Springer International Publishing AG Switzerland is part of Springer Science+Business Media (www.springer.com)

For Ana, Mimi, Laki, Luki, and the relentless pursuit of MSA.

Preface

About a year ago, a patient walked into my office with a history of having undergone a one-sided four-level radiofrequency procedure for lumbar facet joint pain. When asked, he said that he had never had a medial branch block or a facet joint injection prior to the radiofrequency procedure. He had never even *heard* of a pain diary. The four-level radiofrequency rhizotomy procedure had taken approximately 15–20 min to complete and of course it did not help him at all. In the twenty-first century, I wondered how this could have happened. How could the standards of evidence-based medicine be so willfully disregarded? Was it expedience, ignorance, or both? And to make matters more troubling, and what will likely come as no surprise to the reader, is that his case is not unique in having been substandard of care. Further, when put to the test, all too many doctors don't know when they are practicing evidence-based medicine and when they are practicing out of simple dogma. Certainly there are times when evidence-based medicine does not have an answer to our patients' needs or when the answer is not in our patients' interests, but in these times, it is our duty to explain to our patients what treatments are evidence based and what treatments are being offered from clinical experience, anecdotal evidence, or even dogma.

Years ago, my colleague Dr. Joseph Herrera and I launched an interdisciplinary journal called *Current Reviews in Musculoskeletal Medicine.* The purpose of this journal was to provide a platform that would help distill the different specialties' literature in order to provide a uniform set of guidelines for patients with various musculoskeletal disorders. The purpose, to put it another way, was to help move us closer to a day when no matter what doctor you walked into—a rheumatologist, neurologist, orthopedist, physiatrist, internist, or neurosurgeon—the care for any given musculoskeletal problem would follow the same algorithm. The journal is still in service towards this goal and there are many other platforms as well. It will come as no surprise to the reader that we are still a long way off from this lofty but ultimately, hopefully, obtainable goal.

If you treat patients with lower back pain or lumbosacral radiculopathies (e.g., sciatica), then you know that your patients will see different diagnostic and treatment paradigms depending on what doctor's office they happen to walk into.

Sometimes this breakdown occurs along specialities with interventional pain management doctors being more likely to inject, surgeons being more likely to operate, neurologists being more likely to medicate, and family practice doctors being more likely to send patients to physical therapy. Sometimes the disparity in care is within one's own specialty and this disparity sometimes seemingly lacks rhyme or reason. For example, the doctor who performed the four-level radiofrequency rhizotomy on my patient without ever having performed a diagnostic block—the same doctor who performed this four-level rhizotomy tour de force in 15–20 min—is in my specialty of physiatry. How do we explain that and, more importantly, how do we stop things like that from happening in the future?

Medicine remains a mix of science and art. As physicians, we all try to stay in the science as much as we can, but sometimes the data points simply aren't there, or are conflicting, for a particular patient's multifaceted problem and so we get pulled into the art of medicine. Every patient deserves a specific diagnostic and treatment algorithm that fits his or her particular needs in a particular given situation. It is fair and appropriate that as healthcare providers, we should all have our individual styles and techniques. Having said that, there needs to be a common base of understood and accepted knowledge we all pull from. With the journal, Dr. Herrera and I tried to offer that for a range of musculoskeletal problems. With this book, I try in as succinct a form as possible to articulate the evidence-based paradigms for treating common spinal pathologies. In the end, whether a patient walks into the office of a neurologist, neurosurgeon, physiatrist, internist, family practitioner, anesthesiologist, orthopedist, or rheumatologist, that patient's problem should be treated and approached in a similar fashion, and when that fashion is deviated from, there should be a reason.

After reading *Non-operative Treatment of the Lumbar Spine*, when you see a patient with a lumbar spine pathology causing back or leg pain, the reader should know what the research tells us and what it doesn't tell us. The physician reader should know—we should all know—when we are acting with our feet firmly in scientific data and when we are treating patients from dogma or clinical intuition. Dogma and intuition has its place, of course, but we should know and be able to distinguish dogma from fact, science from intuition. Knowing this removes the fear and insecurity from what we do, and it allows us to provide the confident, consistent, excellent care that our patients deserve. Let's get started.

Acknowledgments

It is a privilege to have the opportunity to extend a very special thank you to my dear friend and colleague Dr. Zinovy Meyler for his invaluable input and revisions that helped make this book a reality. Without his hard work on this book, it would have been infinitely less valuable and readable. Thank you also to Dr. Eugene Bulkin for his friendship during and after fellowship together and for his help with assembling the pictures for this book. Thank you to Drs. Stuart Kahn and Alexander Lee for their early mentorship and continued support. Thank you to Dr. Marco Funiciello, my friend and colleague, who offers me a daily reminder that excellence in practice is earned one day at a time and that learning and evolving is the one constant. Thank you to Richard Lansing, Kristopher Spring, and Joseph Quatela and all the hard working people at Springer for making this book possible. Finally and emphatically, thank you to my extraordinary wife and colleague, Dr. Ana Bracilovic, and to our remarkable children, Mimi, Laki, and Luki, for giving me their time and endless support throughout this process.

Contents

Part I
Lumbar Spine Subjects

Chapter 1
Clinical Anatomy of the Lumbosacral Spine

A chapter on clinical anatomy of the lumbosacral spine in a book like this can be challenging. On the one hand, if you don't already know that there are five lumbar vertebrae in the lumbar spine, then you are reading the wrong book. On the other hand, if you do know that the L5 dorsal ramus is much longer than the other dorsal rami in the lumbar spine and that it runs along the groove between the sacral ala and the root of the S1 superior articular process [1], then this information will help you with a radiofrequency rhizotomy procedure (which is important if this is a procedure you perform) but not much else. In this chapter, we will attempt to thread that needle, to provide pertinent, high-yield clinical anatomy needed to diagnose and treat pathologies of the lumbar spine without delving into the surgical anatomy needed to perform complex procedures.

The Spine

Whether you are a physician thinking of the spine or a physician explaining the spine to your patient, it is helpful to think of the spine as similar to a mast on a sailboat. The bones, of course, are the mast. The muscles, tendons, and ligaments attaching to the spine are the riggings that attach to the mast. If a mast on a sailboat is not supported by the riggings, then the mast will fall over. The mast, in the end, cannot support its own weight and so it relies on all of the ropes that attach to it to unload it. Similarly, the human spine cannot support its own weight. Therefore, the spine relies on all of the muscles, tendons, and ligaments that attach to it in order to unload the spine so that it can function optimally and stay upright [2]. This is the reason that stretching and strengthening the lumbar stabilizing muscles are so important in treating the back and preventing subsequent injury. The lumbar stabilizing muscles support the spine, and if they are weak, imbalanced, or not integrated maximally, then the spine will experience unnecessary stress and premature degeneration.

G. Cooper, *Non-Operative Treatment of the Lumbar Spine*,
DOI 10.1007/978-3-319-21443-6_1

Bones

The bones of the lumbar spine serve three basic functions. They bear the weight of the spine, protect the neural elements traversing the spinal canal, and they articulate to provide for a great range of movements (flexion, extension, rotation). There are five lumbar vertebrae and the fifth lumbar veretbra articulates with the sacrum (Fig. 1.1). The lowest two lumbar segments, the L4–L5 and the L5–S1, in part because of the biomechanics of the natural lumbar lordosis, support the most weight of the spine and therefore are the most prone to suffering injuries and general degenerative changes [3, 4]. On the sides of the vertebral bodies are the facet joints (technically and more precisely termed zygapophyseal joints). The facet joints are synovial joints. These synovial joints are hinge joints that allow for flexion and resist extension and rotation (Fig. 1.2).

The sacrum is a large triangular bone with five fused segments. At the bottom of the sacrum is the coccyx (tail). When a person sits, she puts pressure on the sacrococcygeal junction. The sacrum translates the forces of the upper bodies to the legs via the sacroiliac joint. There is some degree of controversy as to the precise nature of the sacroiliac joint itself. Part of the sacroiliac joint contains cartilage and resembles a synovial joint. Part of the sacroiliac joint is a syndesmosis, which is a joining of two bones that does not satisfy the anatomic definition of a synovial joint. In the end,

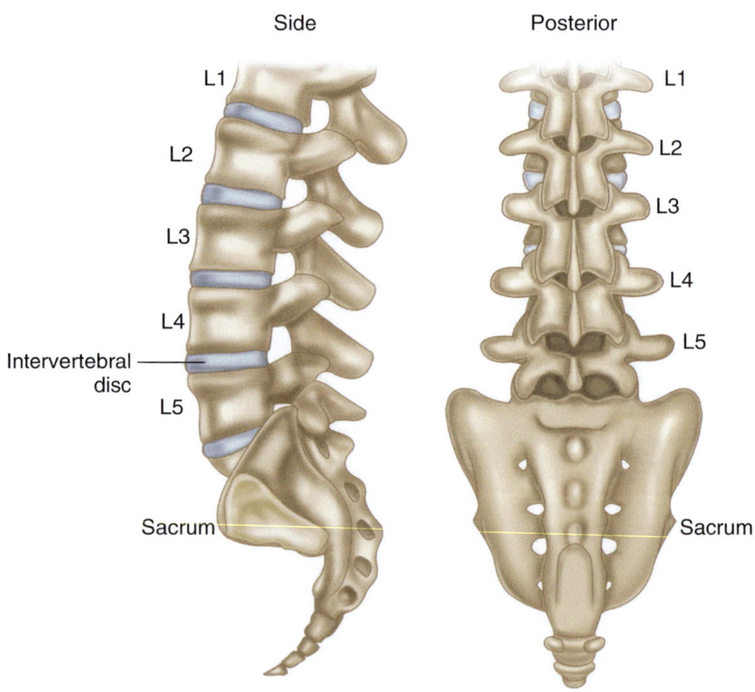

Fig. 1.1 Schematic depiction of the lumbosacral spine with lumbar vertebrae numbering nomenclature

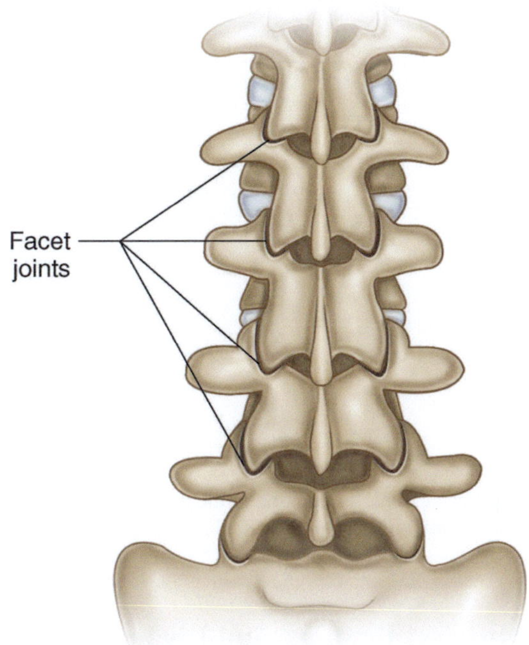

Fig. 1.2 Schematic depiction of the lumbosacral spine with facet joints identified

what can be said is that the sacroiliac joint is a tough, fibrous, stable joint that has some limited but important movement [5].

Intervertebral Discs

Between each lumbar vertebra, and between the L5 and the S1 bones, is an intervertebral disc (Fig. 1.3). It is helpful to think of the intervertebral disc as similar to a jelly donut. There is the inner jelly called the nucleus pulposus. The nucleus pulposus is composed of type II collagen and a mucoprotein gel with numerous proteins with pro-inflammatory properties [6]. The nucleus pulposus provides the cushioning of the disc [7]. The crust of the disc is called the annulus fibrosus. The annulus fibrosus is a tough, fibrous cartilage composed of type I collagen that provides the stability of the disc. In the outer third of the annulus fibrosus, and sometimes the outer 2/3 of the annulus fibrosus, there are sensory nerve fibers [8]. This is a particularly important fact when considering discogenic lower back pain in which a tear extends from the nucleus pulposus to the outer third or two thirds of the annulus fibrosus. This tear allows the proteins with inflammatory properties to reach the nerve fibers, which in turn are capable of causing pain [9]. This will naturally be discussed in detail in the chapter on discogenic lower back pain.

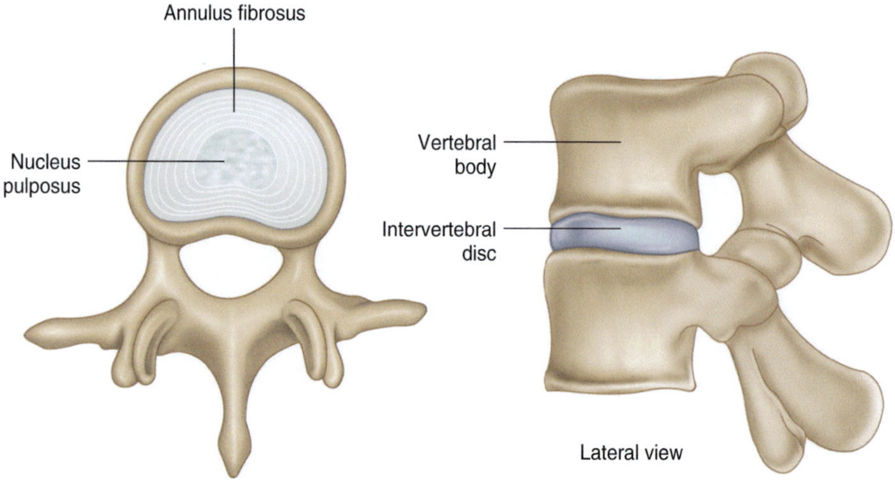

Fig. 1.3 Schematic depiction of the lumbar intervertebral disc, including the annulus fibrosis and nucleus pulpous, and the disc's relationship with the adjacent vertebral bodies

Muscles, Tendons, and Ligaments

There are many interconnected muscles, tendons, and ligaments (Fig. 1.4). The anterior longitudinal ligament runs along the ventral aspect of the lumbar vertebral bodies and discs and limits extension. The posterior longitudinal ligament runs along the posterior surface of the vertebral bodies and discs and limits flexion. The ligamentum flavum is a large ligament that forms the posterior wall of the vertebral canal [10]. When this ligament becomes arthritic, it sometimes hypertrophies and/or buckles contributing to spinal stenosis. The iliolumbar ligament connects from the tip of the L5 transverse process to the iliac crest, helping to stabilize the lumbosacral segment.

The muscles of the lumbar spine flex, extend, and rotate the spine. Perhaps somewhat counterintuitive, the flexors and rotators of the spine are as – or perhaps more – important to the stability of the spine as the extensors. The transverse abdominis, oblique muscles, and rectus abdominis provide critical stability for the spine and are the muscles that typically provide the most strengthening in lumbar stabilization exercises. Also important are the multifidi and rotators muscles which span several levels and are responsible for segmental stability and motion as well as providing proprioceptive feedback [11].

The iliopsoas muscle is actually a combination of the iliacus and the psoas muscles. These muscles are distinct in the abdomen where they arise but run together at their attachment at the lesser trochanter of the femur. The iliopsoas is one of the strongest skeletal muscles in the body and a powerful flexor of the hip. The psoas muscle originates from the transverse processes of the T12 through L5 vertebral segments [12]. As such, when this muscle is tight, it pulls the lumbar spine forward and contributes significantly to increased stress on the lumbar spine. Most exercise programs for lumbar problems involve stretching exercise for the iliopsoas muscle.

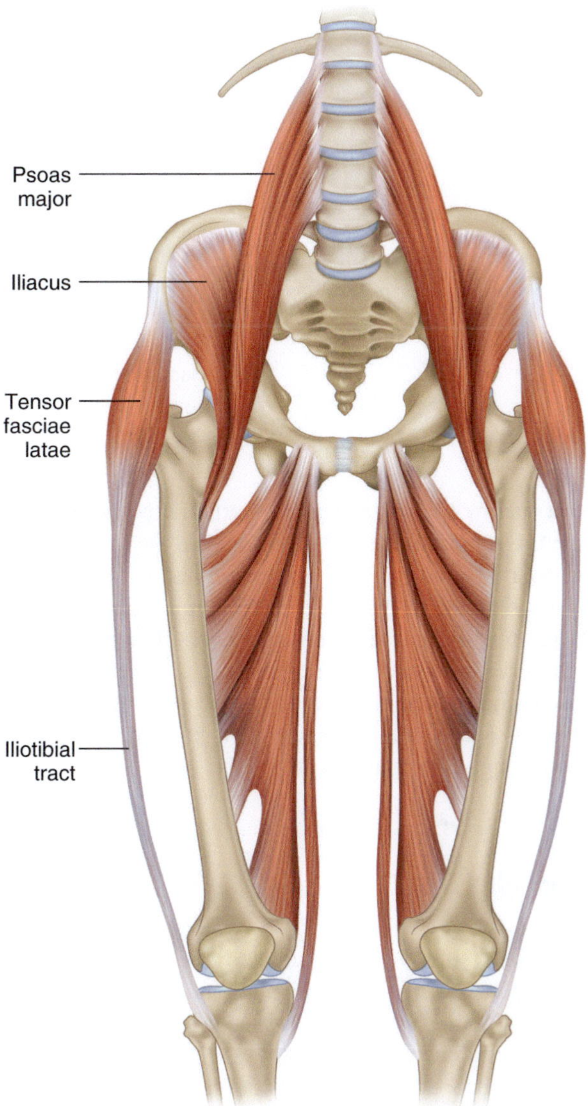

Fig. 1.4 Schematic depiction of the lumbosacral and pelvis with several major muscles, including the major hip flexors depicted

Nerves

The spinal cord usually tapers at the L1 or L2 level at which point it is called the conus medullaris (Fig. 1.5). Sometimes this tapering occurs as high as T12 or as low as L3. At the tapering of the spinal cord, the nerve roots taper out and continue inferiorly within the spinal canal at which point it is called the cauda equina. The nerves exit the spine via the intervertebral foramen. In the lumbar spine, the spinal nerve

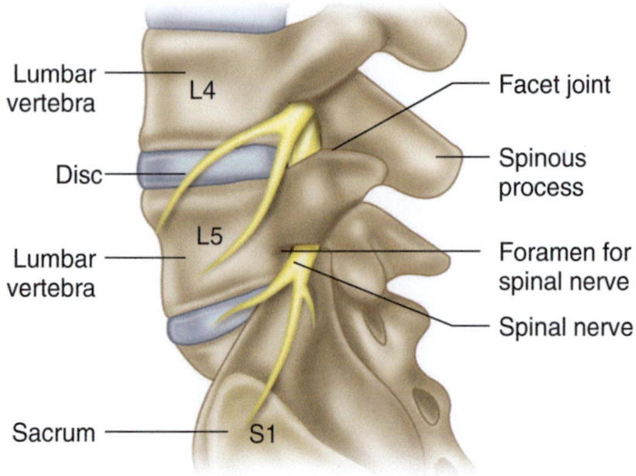

Fig. 1.5 Schematic depiction of the lumbar spine with spinal nerves represented as they exit through the intervertebral foramina formed by the intervertebral disc, vertebral bodies, and the facet joints

exits below the corresponding vertebral body such that the L4 spine nerve exits via the L4–L5 intervertebral foramina and the L5 spinal nerve exits via the L5–S1 intervertebral foramina [13]. The spinal nerve itself is made up of spinal roots which in turn originate from the dorsal column carrying the sensory fibers and the ventral column which carries the motor fibers. Upon exiting the vertebral foramen, the spinal nerve combines with other nerves via the lumbosacral plexus which then give rise to the peripheral nerves. The largest single nerve in the body is the sciatic nerve and this nerve also originates out of the lumbosacral plexus receiving input from the L4 through S3 segments [14].

Vascular

The blood supply of the spinal cord is accomplished by multiple vessels and extensive collateral supply. Some of the notable arteries include the anterior spinal artery which supplies the anterior two thirds of the spinal cord and paired posterior spinal arteries which supply the posterior third of the spinal cord. The lateral columns of the spinal cord are supplied by arterial vasocorona, which are anastomoses between the spinal arteries. This vascular supply is reinforced by segmental arteries which are also referred to as radicular arteries [15]. Venous drainage is accomplished via anterior and posterior spinal veins as well as anterior and posterior radicular veins which largely follow the arterial supply [16].

An important and considered dominant segmental artery (or radicular artery) is called the Artery of Adamkiewicz which traditionally was thought to enter via the left L3 intervertebral foramen. However, as research has repeatedly shown, its origin and side are highly variable [17, 18, 19]. In considering spinal procedures, this artery becomes an important anatomical consideration as obstruction of this artery can lead to significant compromise to the blood supply of the spinal cord (Fig. 1.6).

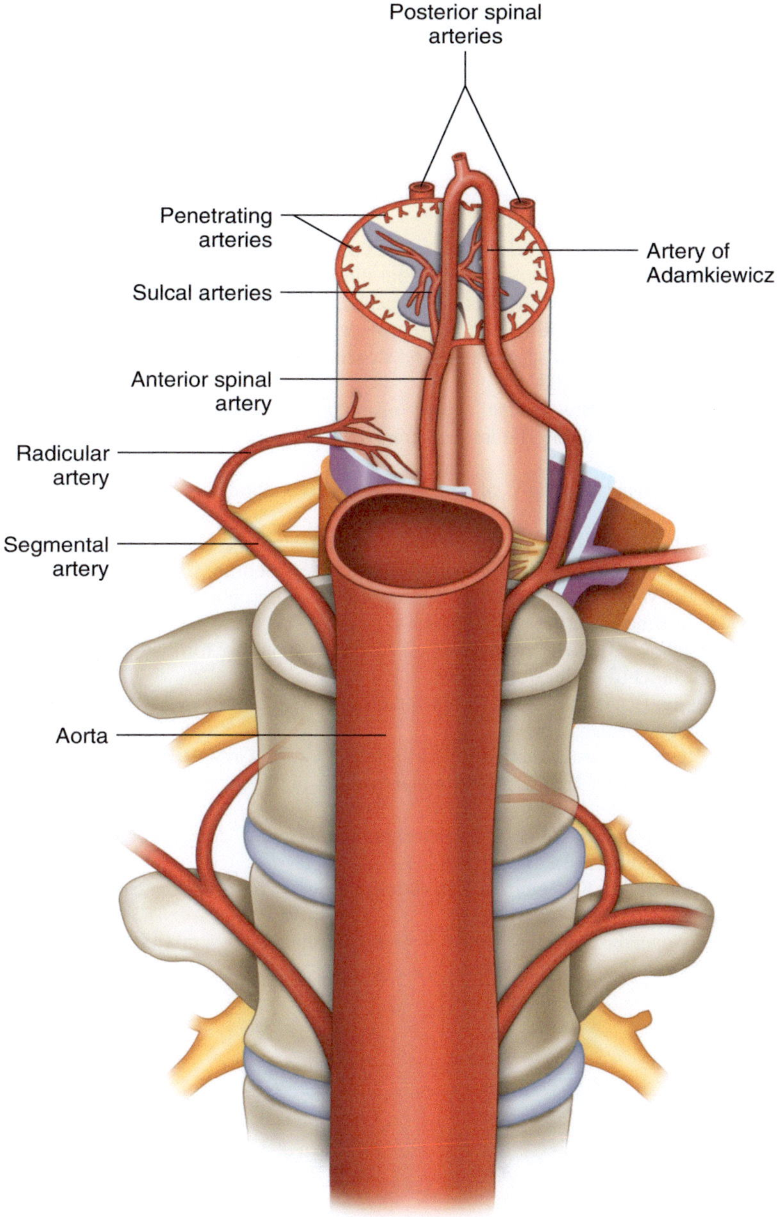

Fig. 1.6 Schematic representation of the arterial supply of the spinal cord and its anatomical relationship to the adjacent structures, specifically the intervertebral foramina

References and Suggested Further Reading

1. Lau P, Mercer S, Govind J, Bogduk N. The surgical anatomy of lumbar medial branch neurotomy (facet denervation). Pain Med. 2004;5(3):290–8.
2. Bogduk N. Clinical anatomy of the lumbar spine and sacrum. 3rd ed. Edinburgh: Churchill Livingstone; 1999.
3. Adams MA, Dolan P. Recent advances in lumbar spinal mechanics and their clinical significance. Clin Biomech. 1995;10:3–19.
4. Adams MA, Hutton WC. The effect of posture on the role of the apophyseal joints in resisting intervertebral compression force. J Bone Joint Surg. 1980;62B:358–62.
5. Vleeming A, Volkers ACW, Snijders CJ, Stoeckhart R. Relation between form and function in the sacroiliac joint. Part II: Biomechanical aspects. Spine. 1990;15:133–5.
6. Naylor A. Intervertebral disc prolapse and degeneration. The biochemical and biophysical approach. Spine. 1976;1:108–14.
7. Naylor A, Shental R. Biochemical aspects of intervertebral discs in ageing and disease (Ch. 14). In: Jayson MIV, editor. The lumbar spine and backache. New York: Grune and Stratton; 1976. p. 317–26.
8. Edgar MA. The nerve supply of the lumbar intervertebral disc. J Bone Joint Surg Br. 2007;89B(9):1135–9.
9. Bogduk N. The lumbar disc and low back pain. Neurosurg Clin N Am. 1991;2:791–806.
10. Williams PL, et al., editors. Gray's anatomy. 38th ed. Edinburgh: Chuchill Livingstone; 1995.
11. Macintosh JE, Valencia F, Bogduk N, Munro RR. The morphology of the lumbar multifidus muscles. Clin Biomech. 1986;1:196–204.
12. Drake R, Vogl W, Mitchell AVM, Mitchell A. Gray's anatomy for medical students. 2nd ed. New York: Churchill Livingstone; 2009.
13. Hall-Craggs ECB. Anatomy as a basis for clinical medicine. 2nd ed. Baltimore: Urban & Schwarzenberg; 1990.
14. Pansky B. Review of gross anatomy. 6th ed. New York: McGraw-Hill Medical; 1996.
15. Crock HV, Yoshizawa H. The blood supply of the lumbar vertebral column. Clin Orthop. 1976;115:6–21.
16. Crock HV, Yoshizawa H, Kame S. Observations on the venous drainage of the human vertebral body. J Bone Joint Surg. 1973;55B:528–33.
17. Parke WW, Gammell K, Rothman RH. Arterial vascularisation of the cauda equine. J Bone Joint Surg. 1981;63A:53–62.
18. Parke WW, Watanabe R. The intrinsic vasculature of the lumbosacral spinal nerve roots. Spine. 1985;10:508–15.

Chapter 2
Lower Back Pain: An Overview of the Most Common Causes

When discussing the causes of lower back pain, it is important to make a distinction between acute, subacute, and chronic lower back pain. Acute lower back pain refers to lower back pain that lasts less than 4 weeks. Subacute lower back pain refers to lower back pain that lasts from 4 to 12 weeks. Chronic lower back pain is lower back pain lasting 12 weeks or longer.

By definition, acute lower back pain is self-limited. Because it lasts so little time, it is generally less well studied than chronic lower back pain. There are a multitude of potential causes of acute lower back pain. The most common causes are thought to be muscle strains, ligament sprains, and tendonitis. However, sometimes spinal causes likely also occur and simply heal in a quick time frame. Because the acute lower back pain is so short lived, it is extremely hard to study both in terms of a diagnosis and also in terms of treatment. Imagine the study that would be required to evaluate the effectiveness of ibuprofen for shortening the duration of acute lower back pain. First, patients would have to be enrolled and randomized immediately into the study before the pain resolved on its own. Second, the number of patients required to witness a difference in clinical response to treatment as opposed to placebo (where the duration being evaluated may be as little as a day of pain) would be huge. And, at the end of it, when the pain is going to resolve anyway, there is not a lot of enthusiasm to run such a large study.

Subacute and chronic lower back pain typically behaves in the same way. The distinction between subacute and chronic pain has largely been made for academic purposes. By the time pain lasts 3 months, it generally needs help to make it go away and it is therefore much more important and easy to study. Because subacute lower back pain behaves so similarly to chronic lower back pain, we will consider them together but should remember that the studies we discuss in this chapter are really on chronic lower back pain and not subacute lower back pain.

What follows now is a brief survey of the most common causes of lower back pain. Each cause will be dealt with in more detail in their respective chapters, but for the purpose of providing context and perspective, they will be surveyed here. There are three most common causes of chronic lower back pain. The most common cause

G. Cooper, *Non-Operative Treatment of the Lumbar Spine*,
DOI 10.1007/978-3-319-21443-6_2

is discogenic lower back pain [1]. Recall from chapter one that the nucleus pulposus is filled with proteins with inflammatory properties and that the outer third (and sometimes outer two thirds) of the annulus fibrosus contains nerve fibers. In discogenic lower back pain, a tear occurs from the nucleus pulposus extending out to the outer third or two thirds of the annulus fibrosus [2]. This tear allows the proteins with inflammatory properties to extravasate out to the nerve fibers, which can irritate those fibers and cause pain.

The second most common cause of chronic lower back pain is facet joint pain [3]. The facet joints are synovial joints and are similar to the other synovial joints in the body. The facet joints (properly termed zygapophyseal joints) can be injured in a number of ways [4, 5]. The capsule of the joint can be torn and the cartilage can degenerate. These changes can lead to inflammation within the joint which leads to pain.

The third most common cause of chronic lower back pain is the sacroiliac (SI) joint [6, 7]. The sacroiliac joint can become painful because of altered biomechanics, trauma, or degenerative changes. The pain ultimately comes because of inflammation within the joint.

Spondylolisthesis is another cause of chronic lower back pain. Spondylolisthesis refers to when the bones have slipped in relation to one another. This slippage can lead to irritation and inflammation, which can lead to pain [8].

A lumbar radiculopathy occurs when the nerves exiting the spine become inflamed. This can occur for a number of reasons. A herniated disc can cause inflammation around a nerve root. Bony spinal stenosis can also lead to inflammation around the nerve root. Lumbar radiculopathies typically cause buttock and leg pain but not lower back pain, per se [9]. However, lower back pain and lumbar radiculopathies often coexist because the same arthritic facet joint that develops a bone spur and causes lower back pain may also create foraminal stenosis and inflame a nerve root leading to a lumbar radiculopathy.

References and Suggested Further Reading

1. Schwarzer AC, Aprill CN, Derby R, Fortin KJ, Kine G, Bogduk N. The prevalence and clinical features of internal disc disruption in patients with chronic low back pain. Spine. 1995;20:1878–83.
2. Bogduk N. The lumbar disc and low back pain. Neurosurg Clin N Am. 1991;2:791–806.
3. Schwarzer AC, Wang S, Bogduk N, McNaught PJ, Laurent R. Prevalence and clinical features of lumbar zygapophysial joint pain: a study in an Australian population with chronic low back pain. Ann Rheum Dis. 1995;54:100–6.
4. Rousselin B, Gires F, Vallee C, Chevrot A. Case report 627. Skeletal Radiol. 1990;19:453–5.
5. Rush J, Griffiths J. Suppurative arthritis of a lumbar facet joint. J Bone Joint Surg. 1989;71B:161–2.
6. Schwarzer AC, Aprill CN, Bogduk N. The sacroiliac joint in chronic low back pain. Spine. 1995;20:31–7.
7. Maigne JY, Aivaliklis A, Pfefer F. Results of sacroiliac joint double block and value of sacroiliac pain provocation tests in 54 patients with low back pain. Spine. 1996;21:1889–92.

8. Grobler LJ, Robertson PA, Novotny JE, et al. Etiology of spondylolisthesis: assessment of the role played by lumbar facet joint morphology. Spine. 1993;18:80–91.
9. Merskey H, Bogduk N, editors. Classification of chronic pain. Descriptions of chronic pain syndromes and definitions of pain terms. 2nd ed. Seattle: IASP Press; 1994.
10. Slipman CW, Derby R, Simeone FA, Mayer TG. Interventional spine an algorithmic approach. Philadelphia: Saunders; 2008.

Chapter 3
Treatment of Acute Lower Back Pain

Acute lower back by definition is self-limited, lasting less than 4 weeks. While acute lower back pain may last up to 4 weeks, in fact it often only lasts less than 1 or 2 weeks. Because of its short duration and relative benign nature, acute lower back pain has received much less attention in the medical literature than chronic lower back pain. There are two very good reasons for this. First, it is very difficult to study something that is only going to last four weeks at most. To measure the effectiveness of any particular intervention would require massive amounts of patients in a study in order to detect whether that intervention was effective. Second, because of its limited duration, testing and treatments are of limited value. Diagnostic testing is rarely performed [1]. Treatments are used to take away symptoms and ideally speed recovery, but invasive treatments tend to be avoided because, again, the pain is going to go away anyway [2].

So understanding that the research is sparse in this arena, what is a physician to do when treating a patient who presents with acute lower back pain?

The first thing to do with a patient with acute lower back pain is to make sure there are no red flag signs or symptoms. Red flag signs or symptoms may indicate a more serious underlying problem such as infection, fracture, spinal cord compression, or underlying cancer. See Table 3.1 for red flag signs and symptoms. Assuming no red flags, how does one approach a patient with acute lower back pain?

Doctors are often asked in training and in board examinations: What is the first diagnostic thing you do when a patient comes in presenting with lower back pain? The answer is uniformly to take a comprehensive history and perform a thorough physical examination. After that, in a patient with simple acute lower back pain, no neurologic signs or symptoms and no red flag signs or symptoms, there is no need for diagnostic imaging studies.

G. Cooper, *Non-Operative Treatment of the Lumbar Spine*,
DOI 10.1007/978-3-319-21443-6_3

Table 3.1 Red flag signs and symptoms

Fever
Chills
Recent unintended weight loss of ten or more pounds
Radiating leg pain
Leg numbness, tingling, or burning
Weakness in the legs
Difficulty with balance
Loss of control or bowel or bladder
History of recent and significant trauma or repetitive trauma that precipitated the pain
Immunodeficiency disease
Immunosuppression such as with a history of prolonged corticosteroid usage
Minor trauma precipitating pain in the setting of a patient with osteoporosis
Lower back pain and stiffness in a young male (20s–30s) who takes >30 min in the morning to be limber enough to get around and then pain that is much more mild during the day

NB: Chapter 14 will discuss the importance and meanings of the red flag signs and symptoms

When considering treatment for acute lower back pain, the first thing to gauge is the severity. If the severity is mild to moderate, then recommendations generally include:

Advice to stay active and continue to move but not to do activities that directly increases pain.

Ice the lower back in the first 48 h after an injury (20 min on, 20 min off) for a few times per day. Heat or ice, or a combination of both for symptom relief after that, with an emphasis on explaining to the patient that it really doesn't "matter" which they use—heat or ice—as neither will affect the long-term duration of the pain and problem and so the patient should use whichever she feels helps her symptoms most.

Over-the-counter pain medications within recommended dosages and assuming no contraindications.

Discussion of the biomechanics of activities of daily living, including education of limiting sitting and proper lifting techniques.

A prescribed topical NSAID (such as Flector patch, Voltaren Gel, of Pennsaid) may be appropriate if the pain is felt to be due to a muscle strain, ligament sprain, or tendonitis.

The above recommendations are appropriate for most patients with acute lower back pain and may suffice for many patients. If the lower back pain is gauged to be moderate to severe, other interventions *may* be appropriate. Some prescription non-steroidal anti-inflammatory drugs (NSAIDs) are (ironically) often safer on the gastrointestinal system than over-the-counter NSAIDs and could be considered. Muscle relaxers could be considered, especially to help the patient sleep at night [3]. If the intensity of the pain is severe, then a short course of tramadol or an opiate may be indicated. The decision to use a short course of muscle relaxers, tramadol, or an opiate should be balanced with the potential side effects. Because they all can produce drowsiness, nighttime usage is generally better tolerated. It is always important to remember that as these medications can cause dizziness, they may be less appropriate in a geriatric population who may already have balance problems and bone density loss. Recall too that in addition to acting on the opiate receptors, tramadol also has properties of serotonin and norepinephrine reuptake inhibition and may have an additive effect with other serotonin reuptake inhibitors such as antidepressants and therefore should be used with extreme caution or avoided altogether in these patients to avoid the potential for serotonin syndrome.

Physical therapy is often prescribed for acute lower back pain [4]. In physical therapy, passive modalities such as ultrasound, electrical stimulation, and soft tissue mobilization can be used. In addition, patients can be taught better biomechanics, and exercises can be performed to strengthen and stretch the appropriate muscles.

Physical therapy has an additional role in acute lower back pain in that it can help teach patients better ergonomics, biomechanics, and a home exercise routine. While acute lower back pain is self-limited, it also predisposes patients to further bouts of acute lower back pain that may ultimately lead to chronic lower back pain. Ideally, patients will look at acute lower back pain as warning signs to take better care of their backs. It may be useful to remind patients that the chance of acute lower back pain returning is significant. The best way to prevent it is to learn better lifting biomechanics, overall ergonomics, and to learn and perform a short targeted set of exercises to help stretch and strengthen the appropriate muscles to prevent future pain cycles.

Many patients with acute lower back pain may also find relief from massage therapy, chiropractic care, or acupuncture.

If the pain is severe and a trigger point is found on physical examination, then another option to consider is a trigger point injection [5]. A trigger point is defined as a taut muscle band that, when palpated, produces pain and also a referral pain pattern as well as restricted range of motion. When a trigger point is palpated, massaging or injecting that trigger point can be very helpful in breaking the pain cycle and releasing the muscle spasm.

A trigger point injection procedure may be done by anatomic palpation or by using an ultrasound for guidance in making sure the needle is placed in the muscle belly. The most important part of a trigger point injection is the mechanical breaking up of the trigger point with the needle. However, the injection can be done using a dry needling technique (in which nothing is injected), using saline to be injected, lidocaine, or a combination of saline, lidocaine, and/or steroid. The advantage of the lidocaine is that the injection procedure is generally less painful. The advantage of the steroid in the injectate is that the steroid acts as an anti-inflammatory and may help with reducing the inflammation from the trigger point and also, perhaps, from reducing the inflammation caused by the injection procedure itself. In this author's experience, trigger point injections can be helpful, and lidocaine is generally good to inject as it makes the procedure less uncomfortable. Depending on the circumstance, steroid may be helpful. However, it is important to understand that there is no proven benefit of steroids, lidocaine, saline, or any other substance injected in trigger points. Indeed, whether or not trigger point injections provide any lasting relief is controversial and based more on clinical experience then compelling scientific data. In particular when treating lower back pain, it is up to the treating physician to use her clinical experience to assess the situation and decide whether this or any other procedure is warranted for acute lower back pain, keeping in mind that none are proven treatments, but all have their clinical place.

References and Suggested Further Reading

1. Chou R, Fu R, Carrino JA, Deyo RA. Imaging strategies for low-back pain: systematic review and meta-analysis. Lancet. 2009;373(9662):463–72.
2. Casazza BA. Diagnosis and treatment of acute low back pain. Am Fam Physician. 2012;85(4):343–50.
3. Hoiriis KT, Pfleger B, McDuffie FC, et al. A randomized clinical trial comparing chiropractic adjustments to muscle relaxants for subacute low back pain. J Manipulative Physiol Ther. 2004;27(6):388–98.
4. Hides JA, Jull GA, Richardson CA. Long-term effects of specific stabilizing exercises for first-episode low back pain. Spine (Phila Pa 1976). 2001;26(11):E243–8.
5. Alvarez DJ, Rockwell PG. Trigger points: diagnosis and management. Am Fam Physician. 2002;65(4):653–60.
6. Institute for Clinical Systems Improvement. Adult low back pain. Bloomington: Institute for Clinical Systems Improvement; 2005.
7. National Guideline Clearinghouse. Listing of guidelines for low back pain. http://www.guidelines.gov. Accessed 29 Dec 2005.
8. Philadelphia Panel evidence-based clinical practice guidelines on selected rehabilitation interventions for low back pain. Phys Ther. 2001;81(10):1641–74.
9. Mehling WE, Gopisetty V, Acree M, Pressman A, Carey T, Goldberg H, et al. Acute low back pain and primary care: how to define recovery and chronification? Spine (Phila Pa 1976). 2011;36(26):2316–23.
10. Cherkin DC, Wheeler KJ, Barlow W, et al. Medication use for low back pain in primary care. Spine. 1998;23(5):607–14.
11. Forseen SE, Corey AS. Clinical decision support and acute low back pain: evidence-based order sets. J Am Coll Radiol. 2012;9(10):704–12.e4

Chapter 4
When Are Imaging Studies Indicated and What Do They Tell Us?

Ordering an X-ray or an MRI can sometimes become reflexive. A patient has lower back pain so an X-ray is ordered. Why is it ordered? What does it hope to detect or rule out? Let us pause for a moment to consider what imaging studies tell us, what they *don't* tell us, and when they should be ordered for disorders of the lumbosacral spine.

Let's start with the basics. Imaging studies give us a picture of the anatomy of the spine, but they *don't* tell us if the pain is coming from that structure. Facet joint arthropathy, degenerative disc disease, and herniated discs that are evident on imaging studies *may* be causing a person's pain, but they may also be incidental findings [1]. Sometimes, the best looking segment on an MRI can be causing the person's pain. As will be discussed in greater detail in subsequent chapters, even in the case of radiographic findings of osteoporotic compression fractures, the pain may be coming from a completely different structure. Imaging studies are important as the best way to visualize the anatomy short of direct visualization during surgery, but their findings must be taken in the context of their inherent limitations, namely, that they show anatomy and not pain.

As discussed in Chap. 3, imaging studies are not indicated in acute lower back pain in the absence of red flag signs or symptoms [1]. If neurologic signs and symptoms are present, then an X-ray is not likely to be useful but an MRI may be indicated. MRI is the best noninvasive way to visualize the spine, including the soft tissues, discs, and nerves [2]. If the patient has a history of cancer or if the patient has a history of spinal surgery at the spinal level in question, then MRI with and without contrast is indicated. CT scans can also show detailed anatomy of the lumbosacral spine but recall that a single CT scan uses significantly more radiation than an X-ray so limiting their use is preferred if possible [3, 4]. A CT myelogram may show better surgical anatomy [5], but the use of CT myelogram, which involves intrathecal injection of contrast and is often painful, is generally limited to presurgical decision-making.

G. Cooper, *Non-Operative Treatment of the Lumbar Spine*,
DOI 10.1007/978-3-319-21443-6_4

If a stress fracture is being considered as part of the diagnosis, then X-rays can be obtained. If a spondylolysis is suspected, then it is important to order oblique X-rays. X-rays may miss acute stress fractures or very mild fractures. Therefore, the absence of a fracture on X-ray does not conclusively rule out a fracture. CT scan and MRI offer better evaluation of the spine for that purpose [6, 7].

If imaging is obtained and a spondylolisthesis is found, then X-ray flexion and extension views of the lumbar spine are often indicated to rule out instability.

If lower back pain has lasted for more than a month and certainly if the lower back pain has lasted for more than 3 months, an MRI is indicated. The MRI helps rule out unusual causes of lower back pain (e.g., tumor) and allows a relatively complete visualization of the underlying anatomy [8]. This visualization can offer clues as to the diagnosis, and it also allows the ability and option of a nonsurgical interventional spine specialist to perform spinal diagnostic and therapeutic injections if indicated because she will have a working understanding of the underlying anatomy before planning the injection procedure.

If red flag signs or symptoms are present, then radiographic imaging is generally indicated, and the type of imaging will depend on the specific red flag sign or symptom. This is discussed in detail in Chap. 14.

References and Suggested Further Reading

1. Chou R, Fu R, Carrino JA, Deyo RA. Imaging strategies for low-back pain: systematic review and meta-analysis. Lancet. 2009;373(9662):463–72.
2. Jarvik JG. Imaging of adults with low back pain in the primary care setting. Neuroimag Clin N Am. 2003;13(2):293–305.
3. Van Unnik JG, Broerse JJ, Geleijns J, et al. Survey of CT techniques and absorbed dose in various Dutch hospitals. Br J Radiol. 1997;70(832):367–71.
4. Brugmans MJ, Buijs WC, Geleijns J, et al. Population exposure to diagnostic use of ionizing radiation in The Netherlands. Health Phys. 2002;82(4):500–9.
5. Al G, Soo MS, Deeb ZL, et al. Degenerative disease of the lumbar spine. Role of CT-myelography in the MR era. Clin Imaging. 1991;15(1):47–55.
6. Jinkins JR, Matthes JC, Sener RN, et al. Spondylolysis, spondylolisthesis, and associated nerve root entrapment in the lumbosacral spine: MR evaluation. Am J Roentgenol. 1992;159(4):799–803.
7. Johnson DW, Farnum GN, Latchaw RE, et al. MR imaging of the pars interarticularis. Am J Roentgenol. 1989;152(2):327–32.
8. Bredella MA, Essary B, Torriani M, Ouellette HA, Palmer WE. Use of FDG-PET in differentiating benign from malignant compression fractures. Skeletal Radiol. 2008;37(5):405–13.
9. Borenstein DG, O'Mara Jr JW, Boden SD, et al. The value of magnetic resonance imaging of the lumbar spine to predict low back pain in asymptomatic subjects: a seven year follow-up study. J Bone Joint Surg Am. 2001;83-A(9):1306–11.
10. Greenberg JO, Schnell RG. Magnetic resonance imaging of the lumbar spine in asymptomatic adults. Cooperative study—American Society of Neuroimaging. J Neuroimag. 1991;1(1):2–7.

Chapter 5
Discogenic Lower Back Pain

The intervertebral disc is the most common source of chronic lower back pain accounting for approximately 40 % of all cases [1]. It is important to emphasize from the outset that discogenic lower back pain is not the same thing as a herniated disc. A herniated disc may (and then again may not) irritate a nerve root and cause radicular symptoms [2]. However, a herniated disc in and of itself will not cause isolated lower back pain. If a tear in the disc is also present, then it may cause back pain whether or not a herniation is present.

Recall from Chap. 1 that the intervertebral disc is similar to a jelly donut. The inside jelly of the disc is called the nucleus pulposus. The nucleus pulposus provides the disc with its shock-absorbing capacity, but it is also filled with proteins with inflammatory properties [3]. The outside crust of the disc is called the annulus fibrosus. In the outer third, and sometimes the outer two thirds of the annulus fibrosus, there are sensory nerve fibers. When discs cause lower back pain, it is because a tear has extended from the nucleus pulposus into the outer third (or possibly two thirds) of the annulus fibrosus, and inflammatory proteins have oozed out and are irritating the sensory nerve fibers in the outer annulus [4] (Fig. 5.1).

Positions that put more pressure on the disc tend to increase discogenic lower back pain. In 1976, Dr. Nachemson evaluated the disc pressure in vivo in patients in various positions [5]. The results were largely confirmed by Dr. Wilke in 1999 [6, 7]. The two positions with the largest amount of pressure on the disc is sitting and bending forward and standing and bending forward at about 30° of flexion. Sitting in general also increases the pressure on the disc. This helps explain why patients with discogenic lower back pain often have increased pain with prolonged sitting. It also helps explain why so many patients report increased pain or onset of pain with otherwise seemingly innocuous activities such as opening a window, brushing teeth, or vacuuming. All of these activities involve about 30° of trunk flexion and therefore expose the disc to increased pressures. The increased pressure on the disc presumably irritates the sensory nerve endings that are inflamed in the disc.

In the morning, gravitational and hormonal factors lead to increased swelling in the disc, and therefore increased lower back pain in the morning is also common in

G. Cooper, *Non-Operative Treatment of the Lumbar Spine*,
DOI 10.1007/978-3-319-21443-6_5

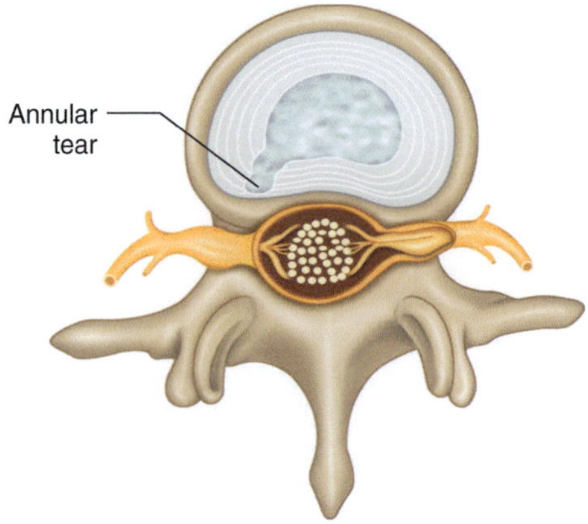

Fig. 5.1 Schematic depiction of an annular tear

patients with discogenic lower back pain. The hormonal factors are due to cortisol fluctuations during the diurnal cycle. The gravitational factors are interesting as they are due to the fact that during the day vertical gravitational forces compress the disc whether the person is sitting or standing. At nighttime, while lying down the gravitational forces are no longer vertical effectively off loading the disc allowing it to expand and fill with fluid. The increased fluid in the disc is minimal in volume but can be clinically meaningful when considering intradiscal pressures in which even small fluctuations can result in increased pain and discomfort in a disc with a symptomatic annular tear.

Positions that take the pressure off of the disc tend to make the back feel better in discogenic lower back pain. This is a guiding principal of McKenzie physical therapy exercises. Extending the lumbar spine decreases the pressure from the disc and therefore tends to relieve back pain in discogenic pain. A common stretch to relieve discogenic lower back pain is to stand with hands on hips and extend the lumbar spine backward (Fig. 5.2). Lying prone and raising oneself to his elbows in order to gently extend the spine is also a common stretch to relieve back pain in discogenic lower back pain (Fig. 5.3). Generally, positions of standing and lying down create lower pressure environments for discs than sitting and bending forward, and so patients with discogenic lower back pain tend to report less pain with lying down and standing as opposed to sitting and bending forward.

Consider the following patient. A 34-year-old male named Jake presents with 6 months of lower back pain that began after lifting a heavy television set. The pain began gradually after lifting the television but then became progressively more intense. The pain does not radiate. The pain is worse with sitting and bending forward. The pain is worse in the morning. The pain is better with standing and extending backward.

If Jake's case were presented to a 100 fellowship-trained spine specialists and asked for a presumptive diagnosis, it would be a safe bet that almost all of them (or perhaps all) would think that discogenic lower back pain were the most likely source of Jake's pain. The interesting—and arguably humbling and depressing—thing is

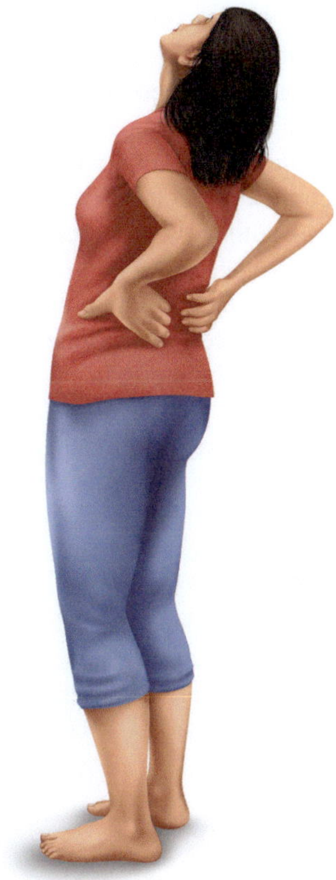

Fig. 5.2 Standing extension stretch

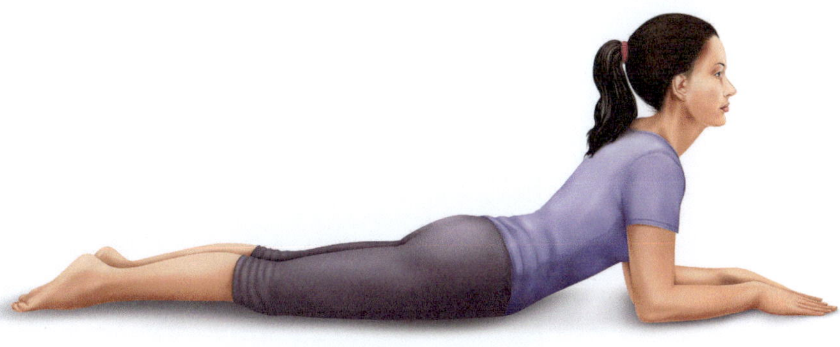

Fig. 5.3 Prone extension stretch

that despite our detailed understanding of the *mechanics* of the disc, despite our collective clinical experience, and despite the dogma out of which we operate, as a scientific matter we have never been able to prove that these clinical features mean that this patient definitely has, or is even significantly more likely to have, discogenic lower back pain. This is a bit astonishing, and most spine doctors *still* are confident that the research has simply not caught up with our clinical expertise (and this author would count himself among that group), but the fact remains that we don't have the scientific data to support the notion that Jake in the above scenario has discogenic lower back pain. If we are being academic in our assessment, then we must cede the point that Jake *may* have discogenic lower back pain, and there is about a 40 % possibility that he does, but he also may have facet joint pain, sacroiliac joint pain, or something else.

The imaging modality of choice for suspected discogenic lower back pain is an MRI. Given the duration and severity of symptoms, an MRI is indicated for Jake. However, an MRI for discogenic lower back pain is of limited ultimate use [8]. MRIs miss a majority of annular tears in disc and, even if an annular tear is present on MRI, it may not be the cause of pain as *asymptomatic* annular tears are not uncommon. With that said, if Jake gets an MRI of the lumbosacral spine and the MRI looks normal except for an L5–S1 annular tear, then it would be hard to convince most spine specialists that this is not the cause of the pain. (See Figs. 5.4 and 5.5 for an example of an L4–L5 annular tear as seen on T2-weighted sagittal and axial images.)

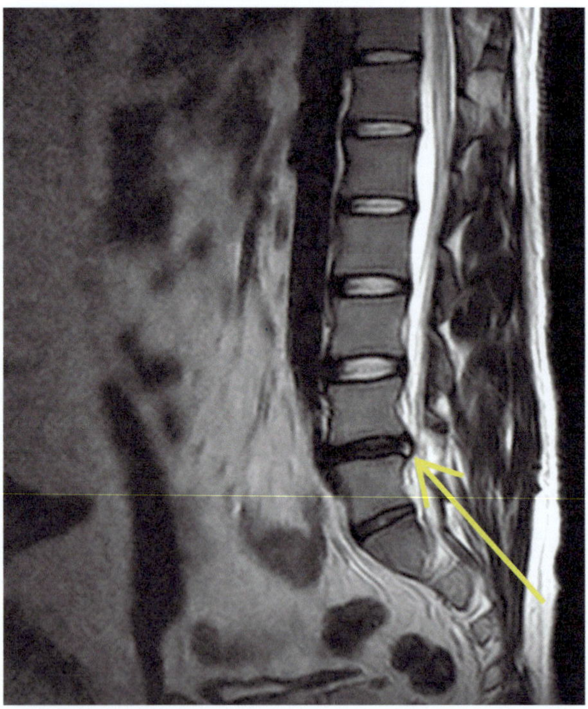

Fig. 5.4 T2-weighted sagittal images of an L4–L5 annular tear

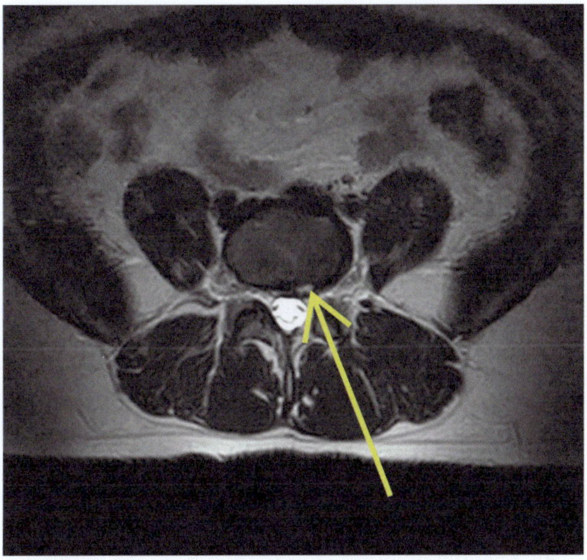

Fig. 5.5 T2-weighted axial images of an L4–L5 annular tear

Though, again, if we reverted to evidence-based medicine, we would have to acknowledge that even in Jake's case, with an annular tear at L5–S1, we still could not draw the conclusion that Jake has discogenic lower back pain. We could posit that Jake *seems* to belong to the 40 % of cases of patients with chronic lower back pain who turn out to have discogenic lower back pain. We could even posit that every indicator confirms that the disc is the source of pain. However, to say that Jake has discogenic lower back pain based on scientific data, we must wait for a paper or series of papers that shows that Jake's features predicts true discogenic lower back pain.

If an MRI is not the gold standard diagnostic for discogenic lower back pain, then what is? For reasons that will become evident, this question will be dealt with after discussing the conservative care for presumptive discogenic lower back pain.

In suspected discogenic lower back pain, the initial treatment is often empiric and based on history, physical examination, and possibly MRI findings. Treatment typically begins with an extension-biased lumbar stabilization physical therapy program with attention given to hip flexor stretching and hip abductor strengthening. In physical therapy, passive modalities such as soft tissue mobilization, ultrasound, and electrical stimulation may be used to help with immediate symptoms.

Oral medications have a limited role on actually reducing the inflammation in an annular tear because very little of the medication actually reaches the disc. Sustained, high-dosage nonsteroidal anti-inflammatory drugs (NSAIDs) may have a role in reducing the inflammation, but at these dosages the adverse effects on the gastrointestinal tract, kidneys, and blood pressure generally outweigh any potential small anti-inflammatory effect at the spine. Similarly, oral steroids are very potent and high dosages may reduce the inflammation in the disc, but the many medical drawbacks of sustained or even short-dosage oral steroids generally outweigh any potential gain. Instead, oral anti-inflammatory medications are generally used for pain reduction. Similarly, muscle relaxers, nerve membrane stabilizing medications, and nonnarcotic as well as narcotic medications all may help with symptom management, and the side effects must be weighed against the benefit for each individual patient.

In some patients, clinical examination may reveal a significant amount of overlying myofascial pain and trigger points in the surrounding musculature. In these patients, trigger point injections may be used for temporary pain relief and symptom management. To the extent that oral medications and trigger point injections help with symptom management and enable patients to engage in an active physical therapy program, they may be considered therapeutic and not just palliative.

If symptoms persist then an epidural steroid injection can be performed. The goal of the epidural steroid injection is to reduce the swelling and inflammation from around the disc. There are three routes of administration of medication in an epidural—caudal, interlaminar, and transforaminal.

In a caudal epidural steroid injection, the medicine is delivered into the epidural space via the sacral hiatus. An advantage of the approach is its relative ease of administration. While fluoroscopy is used, this approach can and is used when fluoroscopy is contraindicated or unavailable for whatever reason. However, because the medicine is starting in the sacrum, a much larger volume of medicine must be used in order to reach the lower lumbar segments, and therefore there is a necessary and significant dilution of the steroid in the solution. Sometimes a catheter is inserted via the sacral hiatus in order to better reach the level of pathology and thus not dilute the medication as much.

The interlaminar epidural steroid injection is another approach. In this procedure, the needle is inserted through the ligamentum flavum using a loss-of-resistance technique. The advantage of the interlaminar approach over the caudal is that the medication can be delivered directly to the lumbar region at the level of the disc and so less volume of medication can be used and a more concentrated steroid can be delivered to the site of pathology. However, because the needle is being advanced posteriorly, there is no guarantee that the medication will reach anteriorly where the medication is intended. Another limitation of the interlaminar epidural steroid injection is that the needle approach must be paramedian, meaning that the needle will be biased to one side or the other. Because of the occasional and unpredictable presence of a thin connective tissue called plica mediana dorsalis separating left and right dorsal aspects of the epidural space, the medication may flow in a significantly biased amount to one side, limiting the spread to the other.

The transforaminal epidural steroid injection is the most technically demanding of the epidural steroid injection procedures, but in many clinical scenarios, it is largely considered the most efficacious. In this procedure, a needle is advanced to the intervertebral foramina around the posterolateral margin of the disc. This is the most ventral approach and therefore allows the most amount of medication to be delivered to the intended site. There are several important considerations with this technique. If there is even a partial vascular flow of the medication due to needle placement, then an intravascular injection may occur. This becomes particularly important if the practitioner is using medication that has particulate matter. Occlusion of a radicular artery due to vascular injection of particulate matter may result in ischemia and its potential sequelae, including the potential for paralysis [9]. Therefore it is important for the physician to confirm the intended flow via live contrast injection that shows appropriate spread of the medication and no vascular uptake. If necessary, the physician should use digital subtraction for added clarity of injection if vascular uptake is at all in question.

Another consideration with the transforaminal approach is the plica mediana dorsalis which may provide a more concentrated unilateral spread of the medication but decreases the potential benefit of diffuse reduction of inflammation at the contralateral side, possibly necessitating the need for a bilateral injection in the case of bilateral symptoms. Ultimately, the primary advantage of the transforaminal approach is a maximum concentrated amount of medication at the site of injection. This is an advantage if the appropriate level is selected for injection, and it also allows the transforaminal approach to be used diagnostically. However, if the symptoms are diffusely spread, or if the appropriate level is not selected, then an alternate mode of injection may be preferred.

When epidural steroid injections are used in presumptive discogenic lower back pain, they are used to temporarily relieve the swelling and inflammation from the disc. By doing this, epidural steroid injections can offer a window of opportunity during which the patient can more effectively perform her therapeutic exercises in order to improve the biomechanics so that the same stresses don't go through the same disc so that the inflammation and pain do not recur. Studies are mixed in terms of efficacy for epidural steroid injections and lower back pain. Most of the studies that have been performed have been retrospective and evaluated caudal and interlaminar epidural steroid injections. Other studies have looked specifically at epidurals for curing lower back pain in the absence of including a structured and rigorous physical therapy program. Epidurals tend to provide good short-term relief from discogenic lower back pain and as such should always be coupled with exercises and appropriate education and lifestyle modifications.

It is time to return to our discussion of the gold standard diagnostic test for discogenic lower back pain. If a patient has pain that is most consistent with discogenic lower back pain; if a patient has failed to respond to conservative care including injections and physical therapy; if the MRI is consistent with discogenic lower back pain (which may mean simply that the MRI is normal, that an annular tear is present, or that the disc appears degenerated); and if the pain is severe enough that surgery is being contemplated, then many physicians will take this as proof enough that the disc is the source of pain and take that diagnosis as conclusive. This would be a mistake. There is at least one more step that should be taken in every patient at this stage. The facet joints and the sacroiliac joints (which are, respectively, the second and third most common sources of chronic lower back pain [10, 11]) should be ruled out as the source of the pain. To do this, a diagnostic injection is performed in each of those joints at different days (this will be described in greater detail in their respective chapters). If the pain is not temporarily relieved from the anesthetic in those joints (or in the nerve supplying those joints in the case of the facet joints), then many physicians will take *that* as proof enough that the disc is the source of pain and consider surgical alternatives to fix it.

At this stage, there is debate as to whether an additional diagnostic test should be performed. The additional diagnostic test to consider is called a provocative disc stimulation test (also called a discography). In this diagnostic study, under fluoroscopy a needle is inserted into the suspected painful disc and also into at least two other surrounding (control) discs. Through the needle, contrast is injected. There is a set of criteria that has been established to be used that evaluates whether the patient's typical pain is reproduced, how much pressure is required to produce that pain, and how many discs reproduce the pain. Essentially if the injection of contrast into the disc reproduces the patient's *characteristic pain* in one or two discs *but not* two control discs and if the reproduction of that pain occurs at low injection pressure, then a CT is obtained after the test. If the CT confirms the presence of an annular tear, then the diagnosis of discogenic lower back pain is confirmed.

In 2008, a multicenter outcome study evaluating provocative disc stimulation was presented at the International Spine Intervention Society that revealed the specific criteria necessary to diagnose a patient with discogenic lower back pain [12]. Using this strict criteria predicted good outcome from fusion surgery. Patients who failed to meet these criteria on provocative disc stimulation predicted poor outcome from fusion surgery. Despite this and other studies, the use of disc stimulation remains controversial, and there are two very good reasons for this ongoing controversy.

The first reason for the controversy is user error. Despite the studies many physicians fail to use the established strict criteria with their disc stimulations studies, and therefore, the predictive value of their studies is greatly compromised. Obviously, this is an area that can be resolved by knowing and conforming to the established criteria. The second reason for the controversy is harder to overcome. In 2009 a study by Dr. Carragee reported that disc stimulation studies may actually accelerate the degeneration of the discs the study is aimed to study [13]. If the only disc being evaluated were the presumed damaged disc, this may be a warranted risk. However, recall that in a disc stimulation study, normal discs are used as controls for the study. Without this crucial aspect of the study, the disc stimulation study would not be predictive (this is an important criterion point in predicting ultimate response to treatment). Therefore, in testing the control discs, the study may actually be damaging them. This remains a contentious point but there is at least some data to suggest it may damage the normal discs. On the other hand, a negative disc stimulation study may save a disc from undergoing unnecessary fusion surgery. Given this, a very careful consideration of the risks and benefits of the procedure must be weighed.

In this author's opinion, a disc stimulation study should be used only when [1] the patient has failed to respond to extended and aggressive conservative care [2], other sources of lower back pain have been ruled out [3], clinically the pain is consistent with discogenic lower back pain, and [4] the pain is severe enough and interfering with the patient's life and activities of daily living enough that if the disc stimulation test were positive, single-level fusion surgery would be performed.

Under those criteria, given the invasiveness and irreversible nature of a fusion surgery, a disc stimulation study seems appropriate. Others would argue that it is an unnecessary extra step and still others may argue it should be performed with greater frequency. And this is why there is controversy which future research will hopefully one day settle.

The gold standard treatment for discogenic lower back pain is fusion surgery. Single-level fusion surgery in patients with confirmed single-level disc disease tends to have good outcomes. A problem and consideration with a fusion surgery is that it takes away the mechanical movement at that spinal level and that means that the movement has to go to the segments above and below the fused level. This raises the specter of adjacent-level disease. The more spinal levels that are fused, the more additional mechanical stress is shifted to the adjacent spinal levels leading to the risk of adjacent-level disease. These risks of fusion surgery need to be factored into the decision-making process, and informed consent process, of whether to fuse or not to fuse.

There are a multitude of intradiscal injection procedures that have been developed. Intradiscal electrothermal annuloplasty (IDET) is a procedure in which a catheter is passed through a needle into the annulus of the disc. The catheter is passed to the annular tear in the disc and then the catheter is heated to 90 °C for 15–17 min. The heat is supposed to denature the nerve fibers in the tear and allow the tear itself to close and heal. There has been some success with this procedure under the right conditions, which are generally young patients with otherwise healthy discs and single-level disc disease [14–17]. However, because the research has been somewhat mixed on its efficacy, IDET is still considered experimental by insurers and therefore is not covered by most insurances [18].

Radiofrequency intradiscal biacuplasty (IDB) is another, newer, intradiscal procedure designed to treat discogenic lower back pain. The concept essentially is that cauterizing the annular tear is the correct approach, but IDET has too many technical factors that make its success rate suspect. IDB was designed as essentially a better mousetrap for the same problem. In IDB, two radiofrequency electrodes are inserted via catheters into the disc and are placed in a bipolar manner. The purpose of this is to denature of the nerve fibers in the annulus as well as to possibly allow the tear to close and heal. Initial results for IDB are tantalizing for select patients with single- or two-level discogenic lower back pain, but the jury is still very much out as to whether the procedure will hold up to placebo-controlled study scrutiny [19, 20]. Until more research is done, IDB remains promising but investigational.

Intradiscal injections of platelet-rich plasma (PRP) to treat discogenic lower back pain is a new approach that does not rely on burning or denaturing the annular tear using cauterization. The idea of PRP being injected into the disc to treat an annular tear is that the PRP may stimulate the body's own healing mechanisms to address the tear. The use of PRP for discogenic lower back pain is interesting and potentially promising, but the research is still in its preliminary stages and so this novel treatment will be explored in greater detail in this book's final chapter on alternative treatments.

References and Suggested Further Reading

1. Schwarzer AC, Aprill CN, Derby R, Fortin J, Kine G, Bogduk N. The prevalence and clinical features of internal disc disruption in patients with chronic low back pain. Spine. 1995; 20:1878–83.
2. Greenberg JO, Schnell RG. Magnetic resonance imaging of the lumbar spine in asymptomatic adults. Cooperative study—American Society of Neuroimaging. J Neuroimaging. 1991; 1(1):2–7.
3. Bogduk N. Clinical anatomy of the lumbar spine and sacrum. 3rd ed. Edinburgh: Churchill Livingstone; 1999.
4. Jaffray D, O'Brien JP. Isolated intervertebral disc resorption: a source of mechanical and inflammatory back pain? Spine. 1986;11:397–401.
5. Nachemson AL. The lumbar spine. An orthopaedic challenge. Spine. 1976;1:59–71.
6. Wilke HJ, Neef P, Caimi M, Hoogland T, Claes LE. New in vivo measurements of pressures in the intervertebral disc in daily life. Spine. 1999;24(8):755–62.
7. Mehling WE, Gopisetty V, Acree M, Pressman A, Carey T, Goldberg H, et al. Acute low back pain and primary care: how to define recovery and chronification? Spine (Phila Pa 1976). 2011;36(26):2316–23.
8. Boden SD, Davis DO, Dina TS, et al. Abnormal magnetic-resonance scans of the lumbar spine in asymptomatic subjects. A prospective investigation. J Bone Joint Surg Am. 1990;72(3): 403–8.
9. Morrisa P, Lyderssa EM. A case of spinal cord infarction following lumbar transforaminal epidural steroid injection: MR imaging and angiographic findings. Am J Neuroradiol. 2009;30:1691–3.
10. Schwarzer AC, Wang S, Bogduk N, McNaught PJ, Laurent R. Prevalence and clinical features of lumbar zygapophysial joint pain: a study in an Australian population with chronic low back pain. Ann Rheum Dis. 1995;54:100–6.
11. Schwarzer AC, Aprill CN, Bogduk N. The sacroiliac joint in chronic low back pain. Spine. 1995;20:31–7.
12. Cooper G, Kahn S, Lutz G, Lutz C, Bast B, Morioka S, Marrinan R, Abbasi A, Tatli T, Berekasvili K, Hyland N. Predictive value of provocative lumbar disc stimulation. In: International spine intervention society, Las Vegas, NV, July 23–25. 2008. p. 174–9.
13. Carragee EJ, Don AS, Hurwitz EL, Cuellar JM, Carrino JA, Herzog R. Does discography cause accelerated progression of degeneration changes in the lumbar disc: a ten-year matched cohort study. Spine (Phila Pa 1976). 2009;34(21):2338–45.
14. McGraw JK, Silber JS. Intradiscal electrothermal therapy for the treatment of discogenic back pain. Appl Radiol. 2001;30:1–6.
15. Liu B, Manos R, Criscitiello A, et al. Clinical factors associated with favorable outcomes using intradiscal electrothermal modulation (IDET). In: 15th annual meeting North American Spine Society, New Orleans. 2000.
16. Bogduk N, Karasek M. Two year follow up of a controlled trial of intradiscal electrothermal annuloplasty for chronic low back pain resulting from internal disc disruption. Spine J. 2002;2:343–50.
17. Lee MS, Cooper G, Lutz GE, et al. Intradiscal electrothermal therapy (IDET) for treatment of chronic lumbar discogenic pain: a minimum 2-year clinical outcome study. Pain Physician. 2003;6:443–8.
18. Freeman BJ. IDET: a critical appraisal of the evidence. Eur Spine J. 2006;15 Suppl 3:S448–57.
19. Kapural L, Vrooman B, Sarwar S, Krizanac-Bengez L, Rauck R, Gilmore C, North J, Mekhail N. Radiofrequency intradiscal biacuplasty for treatment of discogenic lower back pain: a 12-month follow-up. Pain Med. 2015;16(3):425–31.

20. Kapural L, Vrooman B, Sarwar S, Krizanac-Bengez L, Rauck R, Gilmore C, North J, Girgis G, Mekhail N. A randomized, placebo-controlled trial of transdiscal radiofrequency, biacuplasty for treatment of discogenic lower back pain. Pain Med. 2013;14(3):362–73.
21. Tarantino U, Fanucci E, Iundusi R, Celi M, Altobelli S, Gasbarra E, et al. Lumbar spine MRI in upright position for diagnosing acute and chronic low back pain: statistical analysis of morphological changes. J Orthop Traumatol. 2013;14(1):15–22.
22. Slipman CW, Patel RK, Zhang L, et al. Site of symptomatic annular tear and site of low back pain: is there a correlation? Spine. 2001;26:E165–9.
23. Derby R, Howard MW, Grant JM, et al. The ability of pressure-controlled discography to predict surgical and nonsurgical outcomes. Spine. 1999;24:364–71; discussion 371–2.

Chapter 6
Facet Joint Arthropathy

Facet joint pain is the second most common cause of chronic lower back pain, accounting for approximately 15 % of cases in younger patients and approximately 30 % of patients older than 60 [1]. Recall from Chap. 1 that the facet joints are the hinge joints in the spine that allow trunk flexion and resist extension and rotation. Facet joints are synovial joints and as such have the same basic parts as the other mobile joints in the human body such as the knee, shoulder, hip, and finger. For this reason, their technical name in the spine is zygapophyseal joints. However, they will be referred to as facet joints in this book as this is the common accepted medical practice. Pain may occur in the facet joint because of arthritis, cartilage tearing, or capsular tearing.

It is important to recognize at the outset that arthritis of the facet joints is ubiquitous. A cadaveric study that included 647 lumbar cadaveric spines, led by Dr. Eubanks, found that more than half of people between the ages of 20 and 30 reveal facet joint arthritis, and 100 % of people after the age of 60 had facet joint arthritis [2]. From this and other studies, it is clear that imaging studies of patients with suspected facet joint pain must be taken with a grain of salt since asymptomatic arthritic findings are so common [3]. Indeed, the diagnosis of facet joint pain, even in younger patients, cannot be made on imaging alone.

There are features of facet joint pain that are considered "typical" of facet joint arthropathy causing lower back pain. Positions that increase pressure on the facet joints (standing, extending backward) tend to exacerbate facet joint pain, and positions that reduce pressure (sitting, bending forward) tend to decrease pain. Facet joint pain tends to be described by patients as dull and aching. Facet joint pain tends to be more common in patients who participate in extension biased activities (e.g., gymnastics, football) or who are older than 60 years of age.

f the following patient. Elaine is a 66-year-old female with a 2-year history of progressively worsening axial lower back pain. The pain is dull and aching and worse with standing and better with sitting. The pain is worst with prolonged standing still. If she is standing for a while and the pain is getting worse, she says that sitting will make the pain better. The pain does not radiate into the legs. She denies

G. Cooper, *Non-Operative Treatment of the Lumbar Spine*,
DOI 10.1007/978-3-319-21443-6_6

any neurologic symptoms in the legs. On physical examination, she has pain with trunk extension and oblique extension bilaterally. An MRI is obtained, and it is normal except for multilevel facet joint arthropathy that is most pronounced at L4–L5 and L5–S1.

Most spine specialists would agree that it certainly *sounds* like Elaine probably has facet joint pain. As with discogenic pain and other chronic lower back pain diagnoses, this is one of those instances when the research does not line up particularly well with our collective clinical experiences. While mechanically, it makes sense and is consistent that Elaine's pain is probably from facet joint pain, the research suggests that she still may have discogenic lower back pain or another source of her pain [4, 5].

It is fine to treat Elaine conservatively with the presumptive diagnosis of facet joint pain. However, in order to confirm the presence of facet joint pain, it is necessary to perform diagnostic injections. Diagnosing facet joint pain is a topic in which academic medicine sometimes uncomfortably collides with clinical medicine. There are two ways to diagnostically assess a facet joint with an injection. The joint itself can be injected with a fluoroscopically guided intra-articular facet injection. The other injection that can be performed is a diagnostic block of the medial branch of the dorsal ramus that innervates the suspected facet joint. There are advantages and disadvantages to each approach.

Intra-articular facet joint injections are the more common approach of a first diagnostic injection (Fig. 6.1). The advantage of an intra-articular facet joint injection is that steroid can also be used in the injection giving it the potential to be both diagnostic *and potentially* therapeutic. Part of the degenerative process may be a degradation of integrity of the facet joint capsule which may render it effectively incompetent. The problem diagnostically then with an intra-articular injection is that when the medicine is injected into the facet joint, if the capsule is incompetent, some of the medicine may spill over through a leaky facet joint capsule into adjacent structures making the diagnostic assessment less exact. Further, research has not shown that intra-articular facet joint steroid injections have long-term efficacy for treating facet joint pain. Indeed, the research that has been done tends to reveal that facet joint injections work about as well as injecting placebo for providing facet joint pain relief. However, this research tends to strictly assess the efficacy of an injection of the facet joints in isolation [6–13]. As with any joint, if the joint is just injected with steroid, the pain will tend to recur. For this reason, if a steroid injection is performed, it should be viewed as offering the patient a window of opportunity for him to perform physical therapy exercises and improve his biomechanics and ergonomics so that the stresses being placed on the joints are shifted and the pain does not recur when the steroids have ceased being effective.

The advantage of a diagnostic medial branch block is that very little anesthetic is used to block the medial branch and so the medicine does not have the opportunity to "spill over" into adjacent structures (Fig. 6.2). The disadvantage is that there is no significant therapeutic value to the injection (although some studies do suggest a small percentage of patients improving long-term after a medial branch block).

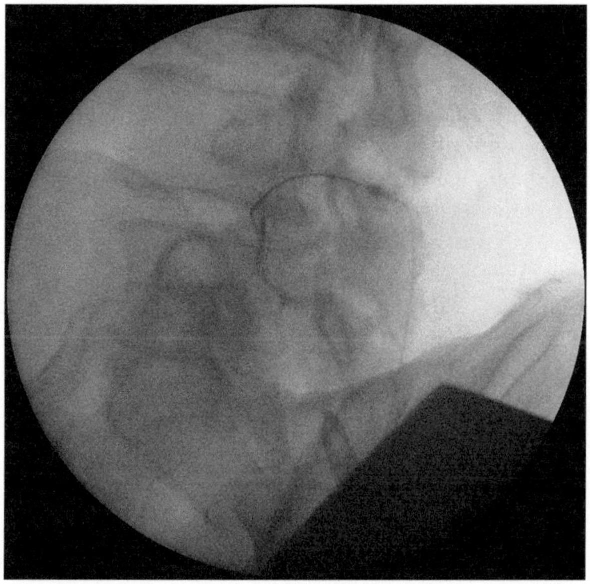

Fig. 6.1 Left oblique fluoroscopic image of a left L4–L5 intra-articular facet joint injection with contrast enhancement confirming the flow along the joint line

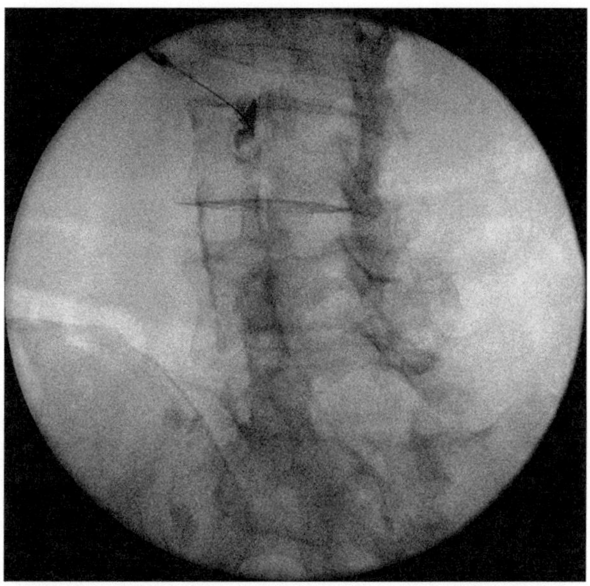

Fig. 6.2 Needle placement at the left L2 medial branch, with contrast enhancement of the junction of the left transverse process and the superior articular process of the L3 vertebra

In clinical practice, the gold standard diagnostic approach to diagnosing facet joint pain is to follow a double-block paradigm [14]. In this approach, the patient undergoes two medial branch block procedures on different days. In one of the blocks, the doctor uses 2 % lidocaine to block the medial branch. In another block, on a different day, the doctor uses 0.25 % bupivacaine. Ideally, neither the doctor nor the patient knows which anesthetic is used on the given day (in the real world the patient typically does not know but for practical reasons the doctor generally does). For the test to be considered positive, the patient should not only have complete pain relief with both blocks, but the pain relief should last for fewer hours using the lidocaine (because it is a shorter-duration anesthetic) than with the bupivacaine.

When performing a diagnostic block of a facet joint (or any other structure), it is important to recognize that complete or near-complete pain relief does not necessarily have to mean that all of the pain is relieved. Rather, a discrete portion of the pain must be completely or nearly completely relieved. It is not unheard of for a patient to have multifactorial pain. It is possible, for example, for a patient to have facet joint pain *and* sacroiliac joint pain. When the facet joint pain is blocked, part of the pain in the lower back may be completely resolved but the buttock pain persists. In this instance, it would be said that the facet joints are responsible for the lower back pain but not the buttock pain and this is still a positive response to the diagnostic test. Alternatively, the lower back pain may be relieved by the diagnostic test, but the upper part of the lower back pain may remain, and this may be due to a different cause such as discogenic back pain. It is therefore very important to explain this to the patient when giving the patient a pain diary to fill out. Another important instruction for the physician to give the patient when explaining a pain diary is that the patient should only concern herself with the response of the patient's typical pain. There may be pain from the needle, but this pain should be ignored as best as possible and the patient should focus on the response of the typical pain.

When performing a diagnostic block, whether a medial branch block or intra-articular facet joint block, it is important to not anesthetize the subcutaneous tissue or overlying muscles. To the extent that pain relief is felt, it is important that it only be felt because the targeted structure was anesthetized and not the overlying tissue. If a 25 gauge needle is used for the procedure, the patient typically can tolerate the procedure very well despite a lack of numbing of the overlying structures.

The reason for two diagnostic blocks of the facet joints is that one diagnostic block yields an approximate 32 % false-positive rate (meaning about a third of patients have a false-positive or placebo response). When the two block paradigm is used as described above, that false-positive rate drops to about 8 %, which is generally deemed acceptable in clinical practice. For research purposes, a third diagnostic block is sometimes used and that diagnostic block is placebo. The three-block paradigm is the true gold standard diagnostic approach for research purposes. In the three-block paradigm, strict double-blind protocol is used, and the patient must have no pain relief with the placebo block, complete relief to the lidocaine, and longer-acting complete relief to the bupivacaine in order to diagnose the pain as positively from the facet joint. While this truly is the gold standard diagnostic for facet joint pain, in clinical practice it is generally not deemed ethical to inject a patient with placebo so the 8 % false-positive rate is considered acceptable [14].

In daily clinical practice, when presented with a patient with suspected facet joint pain in whom an injection is being considered, many spine specialists will start with an intra-articular lidocaine and steroid injection for both diagnostic as well as potentially therapeutic purposes. If the intra-articular diagnostic block is positive but the steroids fail to provide adequate relief or if the pain returns soon after the injection, then the next injection is typically (or should typically be) a medial branch diagnostic block. If the medial branch block is positive, some physicians will perform a third diagnostic block in which the medial branch block is repeated using a different type of anesthetic (lidocaine vs. bupivacaine depending on which anesthetic was used in the first medial branch block).

As was alluded to before, not all patients with suspected facet joint pain require any injections at all. If the facet joint is suspected as the cause of pain, physical therapy is often the first-line treatment. As with addressing other causes of lower back pain, physical therapy for facet joint pain focuses on lumbar stabilization exercises. Often there is a flexion-biased lumbar stabilization exercise program as part of the physical therapy. Special attention is often placed on stretching the hip flexors and knee extensors if they are tight. Passive modalities can and often are employed including soft tissue mobilization, ultrasound, and electrical stimulation. If overlying trigger points are identified in the muscles that are limiting participation with physical therapy, some spine specialists will consider performing trigger point injections.

If the pain is persistent or if the pain is severe and limiting a patient's ability to participate with physical therapy despite the above, then as mentioned previously in this chapter, an intra-articular lidocaine and steroid injection is often used in order to both help confirm the diagnosis and also take away the pain and inflammation. If the pain is alleviated, the patient will often be sent to physical therapy to focus on exercises to help prevent the pain from recurring.

If the pain is persistent despite exercises, physical therapy, and a steroid injection and if the diagnosis is confirmed via medial branch blocks, then the gold standard treatment for facet joint pain is not surgery but rather radiofrequency rhizotomy [15–17]. Radiofrequency rhizotomy is a procedure in which radiofrequency energy is utilized to denature the medial branches supplying the facet joint (Figs. 6.3 and 6.4). Radiofrequency energy is a safe energy source that can be used even in most patients with implanted devices such as pacemakers and spinal cord stimulators. However, it is always necessary to check with the manufacturer of the implantable device to be certain of any precautions or potential contraindications. Radiofrequency rhizotomy is essentially a high-frequency oscillating current that generates heat at the target site. The result of the procedure, when successful, is similar to cutting the phone line. The facet joint may be trying to call the brain to let the brain know about the pain, but the brain won't receive that information because the telephone line has been severed. Without a nerve to inform the brain about the pain, the perception of pain does not occur.

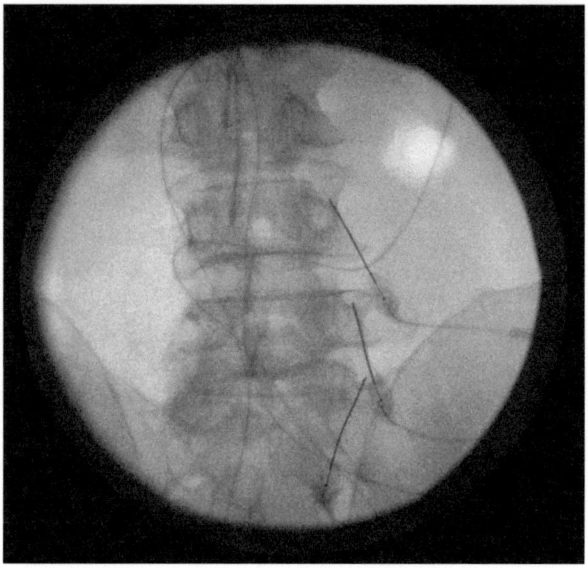

Fig. 6.3 Anteroposterior view of the needle placement at the junction of the transverse process and superior articular process at the right L3 and L4 and junction of the right superior articular process and right sacral ala, for radiofrequency ablation of the medial branches of right L3 and L4 and right L5 dorsal ramus, respectively

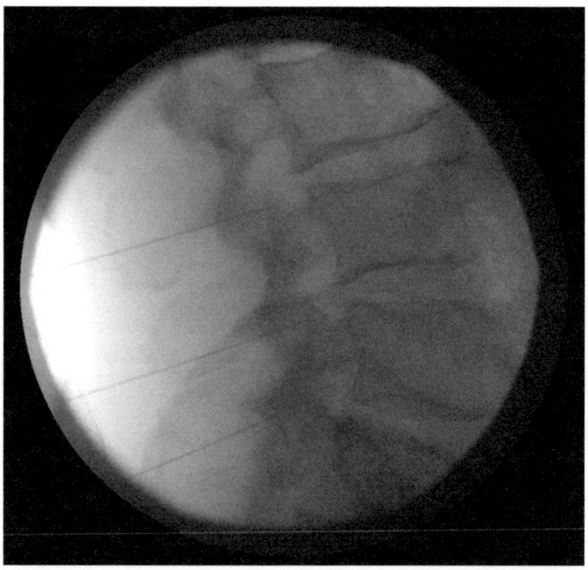

Fig. 6.4 Lateral view of the needle placement at the junction of the transverse process and superior articular process at the right L3 and L4 and junction of the right superior articular process and right sacral ala, for radiofrequency ablation of the medial branches of right L3 and L4 and right L5 dorsal ramus, respectively. Lateral view demonstrates the tip of the needle outside of the intervertebral foramen. The needles are connected to the radiofrequency electrodes, and the electrical wire can be seen in the images

The biggest cause of failure of the radiofrequency rhizotomy procedure in not helping patients is patient selection. When patients are carefully selected with a strict two block paradigm, the procedure is very effective. Early studies of the procedure showed very mixed and often negative results. However, the studies were performed using an outdated procedure in which the radiofrequency electrode was placed perpendicular to the nerve. It is somewhat surprising that a study would show any efficacy at all using this technique because when the electrode is perpendicular to the nerve, the burning portion of the electrode does not approximate the nerve at the burn site and therefore the nerve is often not denatured or only partially denatured. Leaving the electrode perpendicular is easier and more expedient than placing the electrode parallel to the nerve, but it does not achieve denaturing of the nerve. To perform the procedure with an optimal technique, the electrode must be placed in parallel with the medial branch. The larger the lesion at the target site, the more chances there are of denaturing the nerve effectively. Recent studies have shown that the size of the lesion is a function of a combination of several factors including gauge of the needle electrode, duration of the radiofrequency current application, and the target temperature. Naturally, a bigger gauge needle, longer duration and higher target temperature application shall result in a larger lesion. These factors need to be considered within the context of the particular clinical scenario because sometimes there may be factors necessitating changes in one or more variables. For example, a thinner patient with the facet joints closer to the skin may not be able to tolerate a higher temperature because of the potential of a skin burn. In this type of scenario, it may be necessary to decrease the target temperature but increase the duration of the burn. This particular point is more likely to be a factor when considering a radiofrequency rhizotomy for the sacroiliac joint, but it must be considered during any radiofrequency procedure. Because of these technical considerations and because it takes time to properly and safely place the electrode and to perform each burn of the medial branch nerve, any radiofrequency procedure of even two medial branches that only takes less than 10 min should be viewed with extreme skepticism.

The procedure of radiofrequency rhizotomy is generally very well tolerated by the patient. Soreness after the procedure is the most common side effect. Serious side effects are rare and usually due to improper positioning of the electrode. Unfortunately, the medial branch nerve does tend to regenerate. Because of this regeneration, the pain relief tends to last between 6 and 18 months and then the pain starts to recur. If the pain does recur (sometimes it does not and the nerve either never regenerates or else regenerates but the mechanics have shifted and the pain does not recur), then the procedure can be repeated if needed.

Ideally, a successful radiofrequency rhizotomy procedure can be viewed as an extended window of opportunity during which the patient can perform a set of exercises to strengthen the lumbar stabilizing muscles and stretch the hips and hamstrings and ultimately support her spine so that the pain does not recur when/if the medial branch regenerates.

When radiofrequency rhizotomy does not take away the pain (this should be a relatively rare occurrence), but the diagnosis is not in doubt, then it is generally thought that an overlying ligament may have become ossified forming an effective roof over the medial branch nerve and thus partially shielding it from effective ablation; however, it is still allowing the anesthetic from the diagnostic block to penetrate. Another potential reason for failure of the radiofrequency rhizotomy procedure to alleviate the pain may be collateral branches of the nerve that lie outside of the usual medial branch pathway and thus may not be sufficiently ablated but again be in close enough proximity to have had the anesthetic achieve its temporary effect during the diagnostic work up. When this is suspected, then there is another procedure called endoscopic rhizotomy. In this procedure, an endoscopic surgery is performed in which the medial branch and any collateral nerve supply is directly visualized and then cut under minimally invasive conditions. This is a relatively new procedure with little data behind it but good concept rationale. This procedure is still considered experimental by many doctors and insurance companies and coverage for it is unfortunately variable at best.

References and Suggested Further Reading

1. Schwarzer AC, Wang S, Bogduk N, McNaught PJ, Laurent R. Prevalence and clinical features of lumbar zygapophysial joint pain: a study in an Australian population with chronic low back pain. Ann Rheum Dis. 1995;54:100–6.
2. Eubanks JD, Lee MJ, Cassinelli E, Ahn NU. Prevalence of lumbar facet arthrosis and its relationship to age, sex, and race: an anatomic study of cadaveric specimens. Spine. 2007;32(19):2058–62.
3. Abbas J, Hamoud K, Peleg S, May H, Masharawi Y, Cohen H, Hershkovitz I, Peled N. Facet joints arthrosis in normal and stenotic lumbar spines. Spine (Phila Pa 1976). 2011;36(24):E1541–6. doi:10.1097/BRS.0b013e318210c889.
4. Schwarzer AC, APrill CN, Derby R, et al. Clinical features of patients with pain stemming from the lumbar zygapophyseal joints. Is the lumbar facet syndrome a clinical entity? Spine. 1994;19(10):1132–7.
5. Mayer TG, Gatchel RJ, Keelye J, et al. A randomized clinical trial of treatment of lumbar segmental rigidity. Spine. 2004;29(20):2199–205.
6. Schulte TL, Pietilä TA, Heidenreich J, Brock M, Stendel R. Injection therapy of lumbar facet syndrome: a prospective study. Acta Neurochir (Wien). 2006;148(11):1165–72; discussion 1172.
7. Ständer M, März U, Steude U, Tonn JC. The facet syndrome: frequent cause of chronic backaches [German]. MMW Fortschr Med. 2006;148(43):33–4.
8. Shih C, Lin GY, Yueh KC, Lin JJ. Lumbar zygapophyseal joint injections in patients with chronic lower back pain. J Chin Med Assoc. 2005;68(2):59–64.
9. Maldjian C, Mesgarzadeh M, Tehranzadeh J. Diagnostic and therapeutic features of facet and sacroiliac joint injection. Anatomy, pathophysiology, and technique. Radiol Clin North Am. 1998;36(3):497–508.
10. Falco FJ. Lumbar spine injection procedures in the management of low back pain. Occup Med. 1998;13(1):121–49.
11. Lilius G, Laasonen EM, Myllynen P, Harilainen A, Grönlund G. Lumbar facet joint syndrome. A randomised clinical trial. J Bone Joint Surg Br. 1989;71(4):681–4.
12. Slipman CW, Bhat AL, Gilchrist RV, et al. A critical review of the evidence for the use of zygapophysial injections and radiofrequency denervation in the treatment of low back pain. Spine J. 2003;3(4):310–6.

13. Bogduk N. International Spinal Injection Society guidelines for the performance of spinal injection procedures. Part 1: Zygapophysial joint blocks. Clin J Pain. 1998;13(4):285–302.
14. Schwarzer AC, April CN, Derby R, Fortin J, Kine G, Bogduk N. The false positive rate of uncontrolled diagnostic blocks of the lumbar zygapophyseal joints. Pain. 1994;58:195–200.
15. Dreyfuss P, Halbrook B, Pauza K, et al. Lumbar radiofrequency neurotomy for chronic zygapophysial joint pain: a pilot study using dual medial branch blocks. ISIS Sci Newsl. 1999;3(2):13–33.
16. van Wijk RM, Geurts JW, Wynne HJ, et al. Radiofrequency denervation of lumbar facet joints in the treatment of chronic low back pain: a randomized, double-blind, sham lesion-controlled trial. Clin J Pain. 2005;21(4):335–44.
17. Hooten WM, Martin DP, Huntoon MA. Radiofrequency neurotomy for low back pain: evidence-based procedural guidelines. Pain Med. 2005;6(2):129–38.
18. Dreyfuss P, Halbrook B, Pauza K, et al. Efficacy and validity of radiofrequency neurotomy for chronic lumbar zygapophysial joint pain. Spine. 2000;25(10):1270–7.
19. North RB, Han M, Zahurak M, et al. Radiofrequency lumbar facet denervation: analysis of prognostic factors. Pain. 1994;57:77–83.

Chapter 7
Sacroiliac Joint Pain

Sacroiliac joint pain is the third most common cause of chronic lower back pain, accounting for approximately 10–15 % of cases [1]. Recall from chapter one that the sacroiliac joints are the tough, fibrous, stable joints, with some limited but important movement, that translate the forces from the spine to the pelvis and legs. Sacroiliac joint pain is more common in women and also more common in pregnant women and postpartum in particular. In pregnancy, the hormonal changes lead to increased laxity in the ligaments which is what is thought to make sacroiliac joint pain more common in this patient population.

Positions that increase the pressure on the sacroiliac joint naturally tend to exacerbate sacroiliac joint pain. External rotation of the hip such as in sitting cross-legged often irritates sacroiliac joint pain. Sacroiliac joint pain tends to be felt more in the buttocks than in the lower back, per se. Patients with sacroiliac joint pain tend to be able to point more to their pain as it tends to be more focused and less vague. The pain itself is often described as sharper than facet joint pain.

Consider the following patient: Janet is a 32-year-old marketing executive who presents with 6 months of right buttock pain. When asked where the pain is, she points directly to the right buttock over the sacroiliac joint and says that the pain is worse when she does certain yoga poses that involve external rotation of the hip. She says that the pain does not radiate and she denies any neurologic symptoms. The pain is worse when she transitions from sit to stand. On physical examination, her right sacroiliac joint is very tender. She has a positive Patrick's test in which the left leg is flexed, abducted, externally rotated, and extended and the right buttock pain is reproduced. Her MRI of the LS spine is normal.

Most spine specialists would agree that it *sounds* like Janet is experiencing sacroiliac joint pain. As with discogenic and facet joint lower back pain, sacroiliac joint pain is ultimately suspected based on history, physical examination, and the presence of relatively benign imaging studies, but it is ultimately diagnosed using fluoroscopically guided diagnostic blocks of the sacroiliac joint [2–5]. Even an X-ray of the sacroiliac joint that reveals sclerosis or fusion may be suggestive of sacroiliac joint pain but is not diagnostic. Dedicated MRI or CT of the sacroiliac joint is rarely

G. Cooper, *Non-Operative Treatment of the Lumbar Spine*,
DOI 10.1007/978-3-319-21443-6_7

performed under normal circumstances because findings on these studies cannot diagnose pain as originating from the sacroiliac joints. X-rays of the sacroiliac joints are generally limited to trying to diagnose or exclude spondyloarthropathies such as ankylosing spondylitis.

While sacroiliac joint pain is generally located in the buttock and is generally confined to the buttock, it may present as pain in the lower back and it has been documented to refer as far down as the foot. Additionally, other causes of chronic lower back pain often present as isolated buttock pain. Therefore, pain located and confined to the buttock suggests sacroiliac joint pain but does not at all confirm it. Reciprocally, lower back pain that refers into the foot at first glance would not appear to be originating from the sacroiliac joint but the diagnosis cannot be excluded and must be considered in the differential diagnosis.

In order to confirm or refute the presence of sacroiliac joint pain, a fluoroscopically guided diagnostic injection of the joint is necessary [6] (Fig. 7.1). When performed, the injection is typically performed with the dual purpose of diagnosis and therapeutics. The anesthetic is the diagnostic piece of the injection. For a few hours after the injection, the pain should be 80–100 % relieved. As with other diagnostic injections, it is important to remember that a person's pain may be multifactorial. For the diagnostic test to be positive, 80–100 % of one region of the person's pain should feel better. If a sacroiliac joint injection alleviates the buttock pain but not the lower back pain, then it can be said that the sacroiliac joint is responsible for the buttock pain but not the lower back pain, in which case an alternate diagnosis should be sought for the lower back. All too often, a patient reports that the pain "didn't get better" when if questioned more carefully, what that patient would say is that one component of the pain was relieved but another piece did not and so overall the patient may not have felt better. If this is the case, it is important to recognize it so that the other components of the pain can be identified and so that the sacroiliac joint is also addressed.

The research on diagnostic blocks of the sacroiliac joint is not as complete as it is with facet joints. Many physicians accept a single positive block as confirmation of sacroiliac joint pain. To approximate a gold standard diagnostic, it would be ideal to block the sacroiliac joint in the same way that the medial branches of the facet joints are blocked to confirm a diagnosis. Ideally, then, the sacroiliac joint would be blocked on at least two separate occasions, once with lidocaine and once with bupivacaine. To be considered positively diagnostic for sacroiliac joint pain, the patient should have longer-acting relief from the bupivacaine than the lidocaine. However, there is a problem with this approach.

When blocking the facet joints, it is the medial branch nerves that are actually blocked. Unlike the facet joints where the medial branch nerves supplying the sensory innervations to the facet joints follow a predictable anatomical path where they can be reliably blocked, the sensory innervations to the sacroiliac joints are numerous, variable, and unpredictable and therefore cannot be diagnostically blocked. Because of this, in order to diagnostically block the sacroiliac joint, the joint itself must be injected. Ropivacaine, mepivacaine, and bupivacaine have all been shown to be chondrocytoxic dependent on the medication, its concentration, and the time of exposure. It is therefore best to avoid these longer-acting anesthetics in intra-

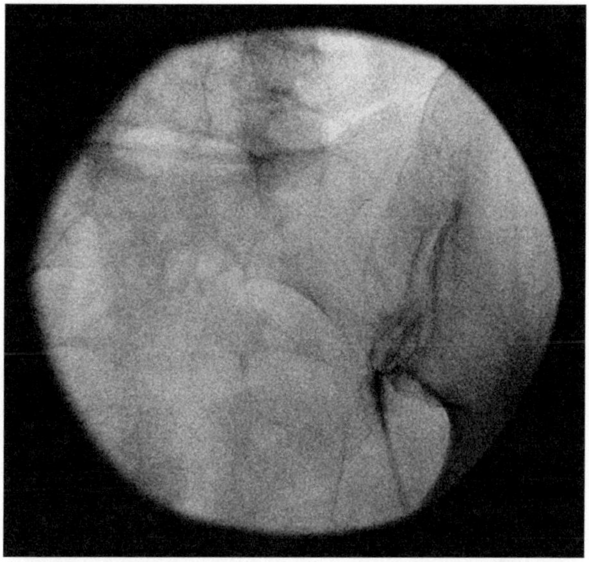

Fig. 7.1 Anteroposterior fluoroscopic image of a right sacroiliac joint injection with contrast enhancement along the joint line

articular injections. Because of this consideration most spine specialists block the sacroiliac joint twice as a diagnostic but use lidocaine each time. Further research will hopefully be done to establish a gold standard diagnostic paradigm. In the meantime, the double-block lidocaine paradigm is a generally accepted standard.

With facet joints, there exists approximately a 32 % false-positive rate from a single diagnostic block and about an 8 % false-positive with two-block (bupivacaine and lidocaine) paradigm [7]. With sacroiliac joints, these studies have not been run with as much specificity, but it is reasonable to infer that if the studies were done, they would look more or less similar in terms of false positives as with facet joint blocks.

As with facet joints, the gold standard diagnostic of sacroiliac joints for research purposes should ideally be the same as with facet joints in which a three-block paradigm is used. In this, in addition to the two-block paradigm, an additional block with saline (placebo) is used and during this block the patient must not experience any pain relief. In all of these blocks, the physician and patient should be blinded as to which injectate is used. In clinical practice, it is considered unethical to inject placebo and it would be impractical in any event.

Initial treatment for suspected sacroiliac joint pain does not necessarily need to include injections. Suspected sacroiliac joint pain may be and often is treated with physical therapy to focus on lumbar stabilization, pelvic tilts, hip abductor strengthening, and generally addressing any muscle imbalances. Passive modalities such as soft tissue mobilization, ultrasound, and electrical stimulation is often used to help reduce the inflammation and swelling around the joint. If there are superimposed trigger points in the muscles around the sacroiliac joint that are impeding a patient's progress or ability to participate with physical therapy, then a trigger point injection may be considered.

If symptoms persist, or if symptoms are too severe to participate with physical therapy, then a fluoroscopically guided sacroiliac joint injection may be used both for diagnostic and therapeutic purposes. If the lidocaine in an injection immediately takes away the pain, presumably confirming the diagnosis, and then the steroid takes away the pain in a few days, then the patient may return to her exercises and physical therapy. Ideally, the sacroiliac joint injection is used to reduce the swelling, inflammation, and pain from the sacroiliac joint, and this can be used as a window of opportunity to allow the patient to participate more fully with therapeutic exercises.

If the symptoms fail to get better with the steroid injection, or if the symptoms return in a few weeks or months, then the diagnosis is often confirmed through another injection using the double-block paradigm. Once the diagnosis is confirmed, the gold standard therapeutic procedure for sacroiliac joint pain when more conservative measures have failed is radiofrequency rhizotomy. There are multiple approaches to accomplishing the intended outcome of deinnervating the joint. Note that for decades spine specialists have understood that performing a radiofrequency rhizotomy procedure on the sacroiliac joint should eliminate the pain in the same way that it does with a facet joint. However, because there are so many sensory nerves running in so many different unpredictable paths to the sacroiliac joint, it had remained a large, mostly unsolved practical problem and efficacy rates of attempted procedures were quite variable.

In recent years, with the advent of newer technology, the denervation of the sacroiliac joint has become more reliable. Previous techniques have always aimed at interrupting the sensory nerve supplied to the joint. This was accomplished by targeting the "most likely" anatomical locations of the dorsal sensory nerves as they exit the sacral foramina. Inherent in that approach is the potential to miss one or more exiting nerves given the variability of the anatomical path for those nerves in part due to the intricate topography of the sacrum. Newer technology has aimed to take the guess work out of the process and create a thermal barrier between the exiting dorsal sacral nerves and the sacroiliac joint. One of these advents is a single probe with three active electrode sites. This technology in particular engages the electrodes in a preprogrammed sequence creating overlapping spheroid-shaped burn lesions increasing the overall ablation size and therefore increasing the likelihood of effective rhizotomy. The additional benefit of using this technique is arguably decreased time of the procedure and decreased patient discomfort (Fig. 7.2).

If rhizotomy partial but incomplete pain relief is obtained with the rhizotomy targeting the dorsal sacral levels then one must consider a potential contribution of the L4 medial branch and L5 dorsal ramus to the superior aspect of the sacroiliac joint. In these instances, to confirm this anatomical variant, medial branch blocks can be employed, and if double-block paradigm for the medial branches is positive, then medial rhizotomy for those levels should provide the remaining relief.

As with other deinnervation procedures for the facet joints, the most common complication of radiofrequency rhizotomy of the dorsal sacral is soreness after the procedure. In contrast with facet joint rhizotomy, patients are also more likely to develop muscle spasms over the following several days due to the potential

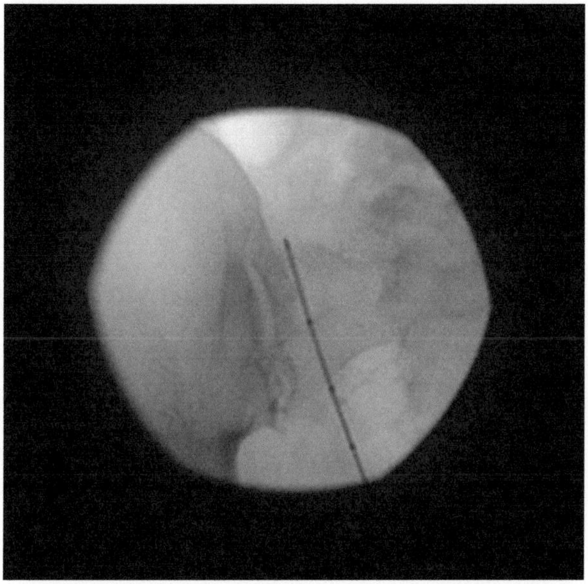

Fig. 7.2 Anteroposterior fluoroscopy image of the Simplicity probe placement along the sacrum, between the left dorsal sacral foramina and the left sacroiliac joint line. Three active electrodes of the Simplicity probe can be seen in the image

collateral impact on the large gluteal muscles. Serious complications are very rare and generally due to improper placement of the needle electrodes affecting the motor function. As with radiofrequency rhizotomy of the facet joints, the sensory nerves innervating the sacroiliac joints do tend to regenerate in 6–18 months at which time if the pain has returned then the procedure can be repeated. Deinnervation of sensory nerves effectively cuts the communication from the sacroiliac joint to the brain such that the brain cannot perceive pain from that joint. When the procedure is done, ideally it can also be seen as a prolonged window of opportunity, much like a steroid injection, during which the patient can focus on exercises to reduce stress that is placed on the sacroiliac joint so that the pain does not recur even if the nerves do regenerate.

As with radiofrequency rhizotomy for facet joints, if radiofrequency rhizotomy for the sacroiliac joints does not provide relief but the diagnosis is not in doubt, then endoscopic rhizotomy may be considered. In this procedure, an endoscopic surgery is performed in which the sensory nerves innervating the sacroiliac joint are directly visualized and then cut under minimally invasive conditions. As with the same procedure for facet joints, this is a relatively new procedure with little data behind it but good concept rationale and as such the procedure is still considered experimental by many doctors and insurance companies and coverage for it is unfortunately variable at best.

Historically, fusion surgery has been attempted for the sacroiliac joint. The trouble with fusion surgery of the sacroiliac joint is that some movement through the sacroiliac joint is necessary for walking and mobility in general. Therefore, when fusion surgeries were performed, patients tended to develop stress fractures in parallel with the joint as the force was translated through other parts of the sacrum.

Newer surgical techniques and materials have sought to resolve the limitations on previous surgeries and reduce complications. Some have reported promising results although more independent research is needed. Fortunately, with the advent of the newer radiofrequency rhizotomy technology as described above, surgery for sacroiliac joint pain is considered a last resort and fewer and fewer patients find themselves having to face that option.

References and Suggested Further Reading

1. Schwarzer AC, Aprill CN, Bogduk N. The sacroiliac joint in chronic low back pain. Spine. 1995;20:31–7.
2. Stuber KJ. Specificity, sensitivity, and predictive values of clinical tests of the sacroiliac joint: a systematic review of the literature. JCCA J Can Chiropr Assoc. 2007;51(1):30–41.
3. Hancock MJ, Maher CG, Latimer J, et al. Systematic review of tests to identify the disc, SIJ or facet joint as the source of low back pain. Eur Spine J. 2007;16(10):1539–50.
4. Slipman CW, Sterenfeld EB, Chou LH, Herzog R, Vresilovic E. The predictive value of provocative sacroiliac joint stress maneuvers in the diagnosis of sacroiliac joint syndrome. Arch Phys Med Rehabil. 1998;79(3):288–92.
5. Dreyfuss P, Dryer S, Griffin J, Hoffman J, Walsh N. Positive sacroiliac screening tests in asymptomatic adults. Spine. 1994;19(10):1138–43.
6. Dreyfuss P, Michaelsen M, Pauza K, McLarty J, Bogduk N. The value of medical history and physical examination in diagnosing sacroiliac joint pain. Spine. 1996;21(22):2594–602.
7. Schwarzer AC, April CN, Derby R, Fortin J, Kine G, Bogduk N. The false positive rate of uncontrolled diagnostic blocks of the lumbar zygapophyseal joints. Pain. 1994;58:195–200.
8. Ikeda R. Innervation of the sacroiliac joint. Macroscopic and histological studies. J Nippon Med Sch. 1991;58:587–96.
9. Bogduk N, McGuirk B. Medical management of acute and chronic low back pain. An evidence-based approach, Pain research and clinical management, vol. 13. Amsterdam: Elsevier; 2002. p. 169–85.
10. Dussault RG, Kaplan PA, Anderson MW. Fluoroscopically-guided sacroiliac joint injections. Radiology. 2000;214(1):273–7.

Chapter 8
Spondylolisthesis

Spondylolisthesis is a condition in which one vertebral body slips in relation to another. There are two common types of spondylolisthesis as it relates to lower back pain and leg pain: degenerative spondylolisthesis and isthmic spondylolisthesis. Other causes of spondylolisthesis include congenital, traumatic, pathologic, and postsurgical [1, 2].

In degenerative spondylolisthesis, the bones gradually start to slip in relation to one another. It is most common in people over age 50, more common in women (by a rate of about 3:1), and it most commonly occurs at L4–L5 [3].

In isthmic spondylolisthesis, a stress fracture in the spine at the bilateral pars interarticularis allows the vertebral bodies to slip in relation to one another. The pars interarticularis is critical to maintaining the integrity of the spinal alignment because it connects the facet joint above to the facet joint below. Recall from chapter one that the facet joints prevent anterior-posterior translation of the bones and so loss of the integrity of this unit allows the bones to start to shift. Isthmic spondylolisthesis most commonly occurs at L5–S1 and is more common in males. Fractures of the pars interarticularis tend to occur in young athletes who participate in sports that involve repetitive extension such as gymnastics, ballet, volleyball, rowing, diving, and football [4]. Approximately 8–15 % of asymptomatic adolescents have been reported to have pars interarticularis stress fracture (spondylolysis) [5]. In adolescents with lower back pain, the incidence of spondylolysis has been reported to be as high as 47 % [6]. For fractures of the pars interarticularis to lead to an isthmic spondylolisthesis, it generally (though not always) involves a bilateral fracture.

The degree of spondylolisthesis is graded based on the degree of slippage of the vertebral bodies (Fig. 8.1):

Grade 1: <25 % slip
Grade 2: 25–50 % slip
Grade 3: 51–74 % slip
Grade 4: 75–100 % percent slip

G. Cooper, *Non-Operative Treatment of the Lumbar Spine*,
DOI 10.1007/978-3-319-21443-6_8

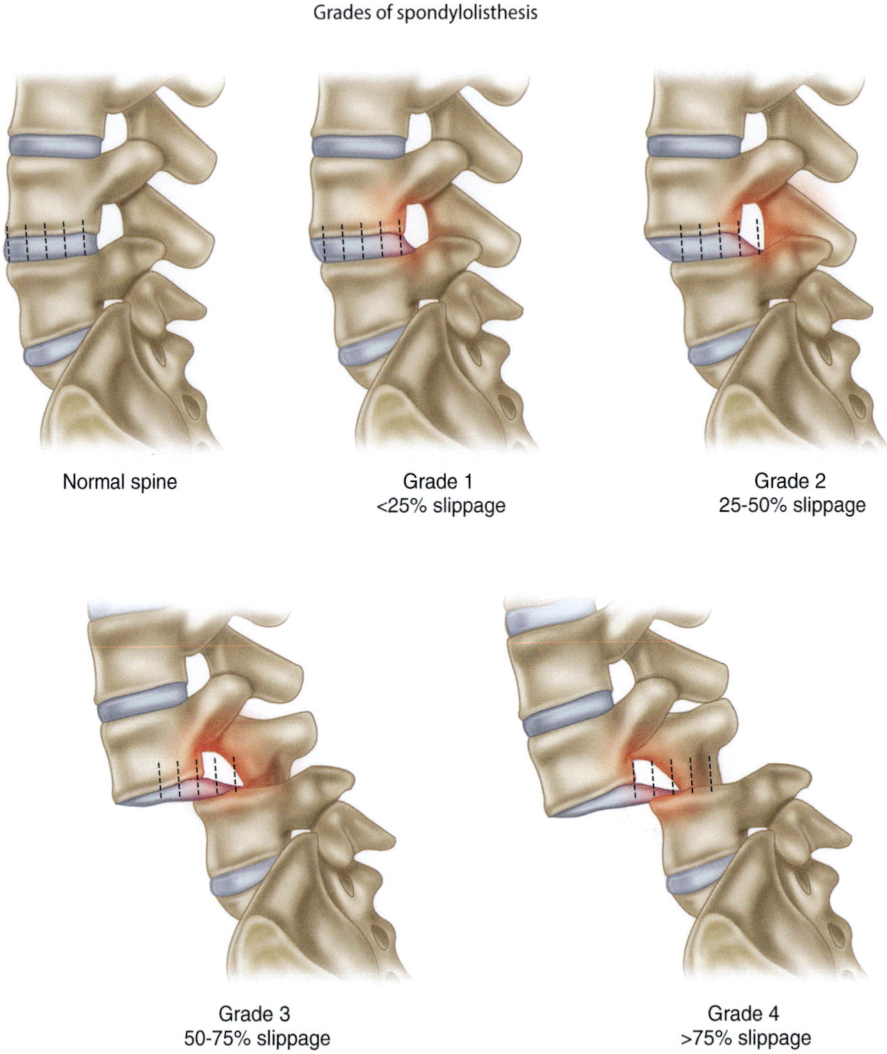

Fig. 8.1 Grades of spondylolisthesis

It is important to realize that *most* people with spondylolisthesis have no symptoms. Some reports estimate that as many as 80 % of people with a spondylolisthesis have no pain [7, 8]. However, spondylolisthesis *can* cause symptoms. When symptomatic, patients generally present with extension-based lower back pain. Sometimes, the pain will radiate into the legs and may be accompanied by radicular symptoms such as numbness, tingling, and/or weakness.

Consider the following patient: Mario is a 68-year-old man who enjoys playing with his grandchildren. He is frustrated because over the last year he has been experiencing increasing lower back pain that is worse with standing and walking and is alleviated with sitting. Mario denies any radiating leg pain or paresthesias in the legs. On physical examination, Mario has lower back pain that is reproduced with trunk extension and bilateral oblique extension. He is neurologically intact on exam.

Most spine specialists would agree at this point in the story that Mario is unlikely to have pain coming from a spondylolisthesis. His pain is certainly *consistent with* spondylolisthesis pain, but epidemiologically it is *much* more likely that he has facet joint pain (based on his symptoms) or discogenic pain (based on the known epidemiology of lower back pain). To complicate matters just a little, even if Mario gets an X-ray that reveals a grade I L4–L5 spondylolisthesis, it is still more likely that his pain is coming from his facet joints or disc based on the aforementioned points. Certainly, it could be argued that if Mario has a spondylolisthesis that this mechanical disadvantage may lead to developing other types of lower back pain, but that is not the same thing as having pain directly from the spondylolisthesis.

Grades I and II spondylolisthesis are very common. Grades III and IV spondylolisthesis are rare (especially in the absence of significant trauma), accounting for less than 2 % of all cases, and an asymptomatic grade III or IV spondylolisthesis is exceedingly rare (though not unheard of). An asymptomatic spondylolisthesis does not require treatment, although grades III and IV asymptomatic cases should be evaluated closely for neurologic compromise and followed for progression of the listhesis or the development of neurologic compromise.

If a spondylolisthesis is present in a symptomatic patient, flexion and extension views of the lumbar spine are often obtained in order to evaluate for movement (instability) of the lumbar spine. If movement is present, this indicates some degree of instability and additional chronic mechanical stresses being placed on the spine and generally indicates a more difficult treatment course. Ultimately, movement on flexion and extension radiographs makes a good physical therapy program all the more important in order to use the muscles to help support the spine.

When a spondylolisthesis is suspected of causing axial lower back pain, initial conservative care is appropriate. Physical therapy that focuses on lumbar stabilization exercises, hip flexor, and knee extensor stretching can be helpful. Physical therapy will sometimes incorporate passive modalities such as soft tissue mobilization, electrical stimulation, and ultrasound to help with the pain and inflammation. If symptoms persist and interventional procedures are being considered, then the first mode of diagnosis and treatment is to rule out the more common causes of symptoms including the disc, facet joint, and sacroiliac joints. These should be systematically interrogated with fluoroscopically guided diagnostic blocks. While the disc is the more common source of pain epidemiologically, it is reasonable to start by blocking the facet joints as this is both a more conservative injection, and, in the presence of a spondylolisthesis, it seems reasonable (though the data here is lacking and so the reader should take this point as conjecture) that it is more common to cause back pain than in patients without a spondylolisthesis.

If other more common causes of lower back pain have been ruled out and the history, physical examination, and imaging studies are consistent with spondylolisthesis causing the pain but the pain is not improving with aggressive conservative care, then surgical alternatives may include a laminectomy but generally involves a fusion surgery in order to stabilize the spine.

When leg symptoms, including pain, numbness, tingling, and/or weakness, is a prominent component of the problem, and spondylolisthesis is present on imaging studies, then the spondylolisthesis is generally contributing to irritation of the affected nerve root. In this instance, treatment involves addressing the resultant radiculopathy. This generally begins as with axial lower back pain with conservative care including physical therapy. If symptoms persist, an epidural steroid injection in which the steroid is delivered to the affected nerve root may be performed. When an injection is used, it is generally coupled with physical therapy with the intent that the injection alleviates the swelling and inflammation around the nerve root and the therapy exercises help support the spine so that the inflammation does not return.

If radicular symptoms persist, as with spondylolisthesis causing only lower back pain, surgical alternatives may include a laminectomy but generally involves fusion surgery in order to stabilize the spine.

References and Suggested Further Reading

1. Kalichman L, Hunter DJ. Diagnosis and conservative management of degenerative lumbar spondylolisthesis. Eur Spine J. 2008;17(3):327–35.
2. Metz LN, Deviren V. Low-grade spondylolisthesis. Neurosurg Clin N Am. 2007;18(2):237–48.
3. Roche MB, Rowe GG. Incidence of separate neural arch and coincident bone variations: a survey of 4200 skeletons. Anat Rec. 1951;109:233–52.
4. Watkins RG. Lumbar disc injury in the athlete. Clin Sports Med. 2002;21(1):147–65, viii.
5. Tallarico RA, Madom IA, Palumbo MA. Spondylolysis and spondylolisthesis in the athlete. Sports Med Arthrosc. 2008;16(1):32–8.
6. Micheli LJ, Wood R. Back pain in young athletes. Arch Pediatr Adolesc Med. 1995;149:15–8.
7. Lonstein JE. Spondylolisthesis in children. Cause, natural history, and management. Spine. 1999;24(24):2640–8.
8. Esses SI, editor. Spondylolisthesis. Textbook of spinal disorders. Philadelphia: Lippincott Williams & Wilkins; 1995. p. 203–13.
9. Sinaki M, Lutness MP, Ilstrup DM, et al. Lumbar spondylolisthesis: retrospective comparison and three-year follow-up of two conservative treatment programs. Arch Phys Med Rehabil. 1989;70(8):594–8.
10. Slipman CW, Derby R, Simeone FA, Mayer TG. Interventional spine an algorithmic approach. Philadelphia: Saunders; 2008.
11. O'Sullivan PB, Phyty GD, Twomey LT, et al. Evaluation of specific stabilizing exercise in the treatment of chronic low back pain with radiologic diagnosis of spondylolysis or spondylolisthesis. Spine. 1997;22:2959–67.

Chapter 9
Spondylolysis

The word spondylolysis is derived from the Greek *spondylos* (vertebra) and *lysis* (break). As the name implies, a spondylolysis is a defect or break in the pars interarticularis. Spondylolysis affects roughly 3–7 % of the general population [1, 2]. Studies have pointed to genetics as possibly playing a role in development of a spondylolysis. While genetics and other factors may have a contributing role, activities that involve repetitive lumbar extension such as wrestling, boxing, rowing, diving, dancing, gymnastics, and throwing place patients at greater risk of developing a spondylolysis [3].

Spondylolysis may occur unilaterally or bilaterally. When a spondylolysis is bilateral, it places patients at significantly increased risk of that patient developing an isthmic spondylolisthesis, which is the most common form of spondylolisthesis (see Chap. 8 for more on this). Spondylolysis most typically involves the L5 segment.

Spondylolysis is thought to be symptomatic in only approximately 20 % of the population with that pathology, meaning that spondylolysis is asymptomatic about 80 % of the time [4]. Spondylolysis causing lower back pain is most common in children and teenagers and is most commonly diagnosed at the ages of 15–16. When symptomatic, the most common complaint is axial lower back pain. A spondylolysis in and of itself will not cause neurologic symptoms. However, if a spondylolysis leads to an isthmic spondylolisthesis, then a radiculopathy may result along with neurologic signs and symptoms.

Consider the following patient. John is a 16-year-old football player with progressively worsening right lower back pain. The pain is worse with standing and twisting to the right. John is a junior in high school and is in the middle of football season. He has been trying to play through the pain but the pain has been getting worse to the point where his coach finally told him that he needs to see the doctor. John denies any radiating leg pain. John denies any numbness, tingling, or burning in the legs. When John sits down during class, he has no pain. The pain has been present for 4 months, since the end of preseason, but has gotten much worse in the last 3 weeks. On physical examination, John is a healthy, muscular 16-year-old with

G. Cooper, *Non-Operative Treatment of the Lumbar Spine*,
DOI 10.1007/978-3-319-21443-6_9

a normal gait and no neurologic deficits. He has pain with lumbar extension and worse pain with right oblique extension of the lumbar spine. He has tenderness of the right lower lumbar paraspinal muscles.

Most spine specialists would agree that given John's age, sport of choice, and extension biased pain, particularly lumbar oblique extension to the side of his pain causing increased pain, it is very important to evaluate John with radiographs for a spondylolysis. There are four imaging modalities to evaluate for a spondylolysis. X-rays, including AP, lateral, and oblique views, can assess a spondylolysis. CT and MRI may be used to detect more subtle defects that X-ray may miss. CT may be more sensitive than MRI for this purpose but it entails the risk of the associated radiation. SPECT scanning is the most sensitive at identifying smaller or more subtle cases of spondylolysis. Additionally, SPECT scans as well as MRI and CT can help identify the acuity of the pars interarticularis fracture and if there is only a stress reaction which may be a precursor to a true fracture [5–12].

Many spine specialists will first order plain films with oblique views of the lumbar spine included in a case such as John. If the X-rays are negative for a pars interarticularis fracture but clinical suspicion is high, then SPECT or MRI may be obtained. If a pars interarticularis is found in conjunction with an isthmic spondylolisthesis, then flexion and extension x-ray views of the lumbar spine should be obtained to rule out instability.

If a patient presents with a high degree of suspicion for a spondylolysis (such as with John) but also presents with neurologic features, then it may be best to order an MRI as this does not include radiation and will also show the soft tissues and potential for concomitant disc herniation or other pathology.

Treatment for a spondylolysis depends on the stage of the fracture. Pain medications, bracing, and rest are the cornerstone of treatments for acute fractures. Pain medications may include acetaminophen, NSAIDs, muscle relaxers, or a short course of opiates depending on the severity of symptoms.

If John were to have been found to have an acute spondylolysis, he would have to abstain from football until he was fully healed and then he would make incremental return to sport. It is safe to say that if John had an acute spondylolysis, his football season would have been over but not necessarily his football career. If John had a spondylolysis, he would likely have been prescribed a Boston overlapping brace to be worn for 23 h per day and he would have been prescribed physical therapy.

Once John was symptom-free for 3 months, a repeat bone scan would be performed. If that revealed bony union or a pain-free fibrous union, then he would be able to progress his physical therapy with a special focus on core strengthening and knee extensor stretching. It is important to remember that a patient who has been braced for any length of time will need extra time to strengthen his core, particularly if that patient is planning to return to sport.

If the fracture in John's case were not healed at 3 months, he may need to continue wearing the brace for several more months. Most acute fractures heal within 3–9 months. Once a fracture is healed, return to full activities (including dance, football, gymnastics, etc.) generally begins about 6 weeks after the patient is pain-free. The patient should be able to demonstrate normal flexibility and good strength.

The return to activity should be gradual and incremental and should not cause a recurrence of the patient's lower back pain. If lower back pain does result from a return to activity, then the activity should be immediately stopped and the patient should return for further evaluation.

In rare cases, the spondylolysis does not heal and the patient may be considered as a surgical candidate. In uncomplicated cases of spondylolysis (e.g., cases without a concomitant isthmic spondylolisthesis or other problem), this should be rare.

It is important to remember that the radiographic finding of a spondylolysis in the presence of lower back pain does not mean that the correlation equals causation. Recall that about 80 % of spondylolysis are asymptomatic. If the clinical case were of a 40-year-old male with a 6-month history of gradually worsening axial lower back pain that was worse with sitting and better with standing, and if this 40-year-old male did not play football or participate in any other at-risk activity, then it would be unlikely (though not impossible) that the spondylolysis were causing his back pain. Indeed, in a situation like this, even in the presence of a radiographic spondylolysis, discogenic lower back pain would still be the most likely diagnosis based on epidemiology alone.

Patients with an asymptomatic isolated spondylolysis do not require treatment. Ideally, a patient with an asymptomatic spondylolysis would participate in lumbar stabilization exercises and knee extensor stretching exercises as part of an overall exercise routine, but this recommendation would be true for all people.

References and Suggested Further Reading

1. Grobler LJ, Wiltse LL. Classification, and nonoperative and operative treatment of spondylolisthesis. In: Frymoyer's the adult spine: principles and practice. 2nd ed. Philadelphia: Lippincott; 1997. p. 1865–921.
2. Beutler WJ, Fredrickson BE, Murtland A, et al. The natural history of spondylolysis and spondylolisthesis: 45-year follow-up evaluation. Spine. 2003;28(10):1027–35; discussion 1035.
3. Zetaruk M. Lumbar spine injuries. In: Micheli LJ, Purcell LK, editors. The adolescent athlete. New York: Springer; 2007. p. 109–40.
4. Logroscino G, Mazza O, Aulisa G, Pitta L, Pola E, Aulisa L. Spondylolysis and spondylolisthesis in the pediatric and adolescent population. Childs Nerv Syst. 2001;17(11):644–55. Epub 2001 Oct 27.
5. Ulmer JL, Mathews VP, Elster AD, et al. MR imaging of lumbar spondylolysis: the importance of ancillary observations. Am J Roentgenol. 1997;169(1):233–9.
6. Ulmer JL, Elster AD, Mathews VP, Allen AM. Lumbar spondylolysis: reactive marrow changes seen in adjacent pedicles on MR images. Am J Roentgenol. 1995;164(2):429–33.
7. Mofidi A, Tansey C, Mahapatra SR, Mirza HA, Eisenstein SM. Cervical spondylolysis, radiologic pointers of stability and acute traumatic as opposed to chronic spondylolysis. J Spinal Disord Tech. 2007;20(6):473–9.
8. Krupski W, Majcher P, Tatara MR. Computed tomography diagnostic of lumbar spondylolysis. Ortop Traumatol Rehabil. 2004;6(5):652–7.
9. Krupski W, Majcher P. Radiological diagnostic of lumbar spondylolysis. Ortop Traumatol Rehabil. 2004;6(6):809–18.

10. Masharawi Y, Dar G, Peleg S, Steinberg N, Alperovitch-Najenson D, Salame K. Lumbar facet anatomy changes in spondylolysis: a comparative skeletal study. Eur Spine J. 2007; 16(7):993–9.
11. Sairyo K, Katoh S, Takata Y, Terai T, Yasui N, Goel VK. MRI signal changes of the pedicle as an indicator for early diagnosis of spondylolysis in children and adolescents: a clinical and biomechanical study. Spine. 2006;31(2):206–11.
12. Gregory PL, Batt ME, Kerslake RW, Webb JK. Single photon emission computerized tomography and reverse gantry computerized tomography findings in patients with back pain investigated for spondylolysis. Clin J Sport Med. 2005;15(2):79–86.
13. Lundin DA, Wiseman DB, Shaffrey CI. Spondylolysis and spondylolisthesis in the athlete. Clin Neurosurg. 2002;49:528–47.
14. Kraft DE. Low back pain in the adolescent athlete. Pediatr Clin North Am. 2002;49(3):643–53.

Chapter 10
Lumbosacral Radiculopathy

A lumbosacral radiculopathy is commonly referred to by patients and doctors alike as a "pinched nerve" or "sciatica." Translated from Latin and Greek, a radiculopathy is simply a pathology (*pathos* from the Greek) of a nerve root (*radix* from the Latin). A true radiculopathy means that there is neurologic loss of the spinal nerve, meaning loss of strength or sensation. A radiculitis refers to inflammation of a spinal nerve and can result in only pain or the subjective sensation of numbness, tingling, or even subjective weakness as opposed to objective loss of sensation or strength on physical examination. For the purposes of this chapter, we will consider a lumbosacral radiculopathy and radiculitis together under the term lumbosacral radiculopathy, meaning impingement and/or inflammation of one or more spinal nerves in the lumbosacral spine.

A lumbosacral radiculopathy may result from many causes. Anything or things that inflames or compresses a nerve root may result in a radiculopathy. The most common of these factors are facet joint arthropathy and/or herniated discs, but a facet joint cyst, scar tissue from a previous surgery, or a buckled ligamentum flavum could also create the conditions that lead to a lumbosacral radiculopathy. In younger patients, an acute herniated disc is more common as a cause. In older patients, a confluence of degenerative spinal factors is more common as a cause.

Common symptoms of a lumbosacral radiculopathy include one or more of the following symptoms: radiating leg pain, numbness, tingling, and weakness. It is important to recognize that while a radiculopathy may be associated with lower back pain, it is not in and of itself a typical direct cause of lower back pain. A herniated disc may inflame or compress a nerve root causing a radiculopathy. However, it is important to remember that a herniated disc may, and commonly does, exist in a person with no symptoms whatsoever. Facet joint arthropathy, facet joint-derived cyst, spondylolisthesis, and ligamentum flavum hypertrophy and buckling all may contribute to foraminal stenosis that may result in a radiculopathy – although again all of these changes may happen in someone who is completely asymptomatic. Often, a disc may cause lower back pain in addition to inflaming a nerve root in

G. Cooper, *Non-Operative Treatment of the Lumbar Spine*,
DOI 10.1007/978-3-319-21443-6_10

which case the pain is multifactorial. Additionally, in the presence of a radiculopathy, the muscles may spasm and guard leading to secondary lower back pain.

Consider the following patient: Anastasia is a 52-year-old violinist who presents with a 3-month history of right lower back pain radiating into the right posterior and lateral thigh and into the posterior and lateral calf and into the lateral and dorsum of the foot and big toe. The pain is described as burning. She sometimes feels numbness in the right foot. She denies any weakness. The pain and numbness is worse with prolonged sitting and better with standing and walking around. She rates the pain as 6/10 on VAS. On physical examination, Anastasia has a positive straight leg raise at 40° and has 4+/5 strength in the right hip abductors, extensor hallucis longus (EHL), and plantar flexors. Otherwise, she is neurologically intact. Her right L4, L5, and S1 paraspinals are tender as is her right quadrates lumborum muscle and piriformis muscle. She has pain at 30° of trunk flexion and feels better with trunk extension, including with oblique trunk extension bilaterally.

Most spine specialists would immediately agree and recognize that Anastasia is suffering from symptoms most consistent with a radiculopathy that is likely affecting her right L5 and S1 spinal nerves. Radiculopathies are relatively common with some estimates of them affecting 1 in 20 people [1]. When there is inflammation along the nerve root, it is not uncommon for the muscles to spasm and/or tighten along the distribution of the nerve. For this reason, the piriformis muscle (as well as muscles in the lower back) is often very tight and tender in patients with L5 and S1 radiculopathies.

A historical common pitfall in the diagnosis of lumbosacral radiculopathies was that the examining physician would press on the piriformis muscle on examination and find that it reproduced some of the patient's pain. A presumptive diagnosis of piriformis syndrome was made followed by an injection of lidocaine and steroid into the piriformis muscle. The injection into the piriformis muscle often led to temporary relief of some of the symptoms leading physicians to label the pain confidently as "piriformis syndrome." However, the pain would typically recur a week or two later because in most cases (>98 %) the piriformis muscle in spasm was a *symptom of the problem* rather than the underlying cause. As our understanding of the spine has evolved, this has become clear and by healing the L5–S1 nerve roots, the piriformis muscle typically relaxes and is no longer symptomatic without ever having to inject it.

A clinical pearl to consider is in the physical examination of the hip abductors. There are two good ways to assess this muscle group. The most gross muscle testing is to have the patient stand on one leg and assess if the patient falls into a Trendelenburg stance because the hip abductors do not support the patient. For more subtle testing, most physicians will have the patient lie on their side and push up, abducting their leg against the physician's resistance. The pearl is to first bring the patient's leg into slight hip extension before testing the abduction. Failing to do this allows the patient to inadvertently use her hip flexors in the testing, and because the flexors are a powerful muscle group, the hip abductor weakness, particularly if it is a subtle weakness, is missed.

When a radiculopathy is suspected, imaging is often indicated. The most common and valuable imaging study to obtain is MRI [2, 3]. It is important to always remember that asymptomatic findings on MRI (e.g., facet joint arthropathy, herniated disc) are common and therefore must be viewed as one piece of the diagnostic puzzle [4]. However, if the findings on the MRI are consistent with the patient's reported symptoms and objective physical examination findings, the diagnosis is typically secured. If the MRI is not consistent with the history and physical examination, then electrodiagnostic studies (EMG/NCS) may be ordered to help determine and secure the diagnosis [5, 6]. Indeed, it is not uncommon for the MRI to be ambiguous or inconsistent with the patient's history and physical examination findings. This point underscores the fact that most radiculopathies are inflammatory in nature rather than a true mechanical compression of a nerve root.

For most patients with a lumbosacral radiculopathy, conservative care is a helpful and appropriate first step of treatment. Physical therapy is often utilized at the outset and this will generally consist of lumbar stabilization exercises, hip stretches, and muscle balancing [7]. Passive modalities such as electrical stimulation, ultrasound, heat, and soft tissue mobilization may also be incorporated. If the pain limits the patient's ability to participate with physical therapy or if physical therapy is not helpful, then a targeted epidural steroid injection may be used. The purpose of the epidural steroid injection is to reduce the swelling and inflammation from around the nerve root [8].

There are three modes of delivery of the steroid in an epidural steroid injection to the epidural space. This was discussed in the chapter on discogenic lower back pain but will be reviewed in this chapter again in case the reader has skipped to this chapter. The three modes of delivery include a caudal epidural steroid injection, interlaminar epidural steroid injection, and a transforaminal epidural steroid injection.

In a caudal epidural steroid injection, the medicine is delivered into the epidural space via the sacral hiatus (Figs. 10.1 and 10.2). An advantage of the approach is its relative ease of administration. While fluoroscopy is used, this approach can and is used when fluoroscopy is contraindicated or unavailable for whatever reason. However, because the medicine is starting in the sacrum, a much larger volume of medicine must be used in order to reach the lower lumbar segments, and therefore, there is a necessary and significant dilution of the steroid in the solution. Sometimes a catheter is inserted via the sacral hiatus in order to better reach the level of pathology and thus not dilute the medication as much.

The interlaminar epidural steroid injection is another approach. In this procedure, the needle is inserted through the ligamentum flavum using a loss-of-resistance technique. The advantage of the interlaminar approach over the caudal is that the medication can be delivered directly to the lumbar region at the level of the disc and so less volume of medication can be used and a more concentrated steroid can be delivered to the site of pathology. However, because the needle is being advanced posteriorly, there is no guarantee that the medication will reach anteriorly where the medication is intended. Another limitation of the interlaminar epidural steroid injection is that the needle approach must be paramedian, meaning that the needle will

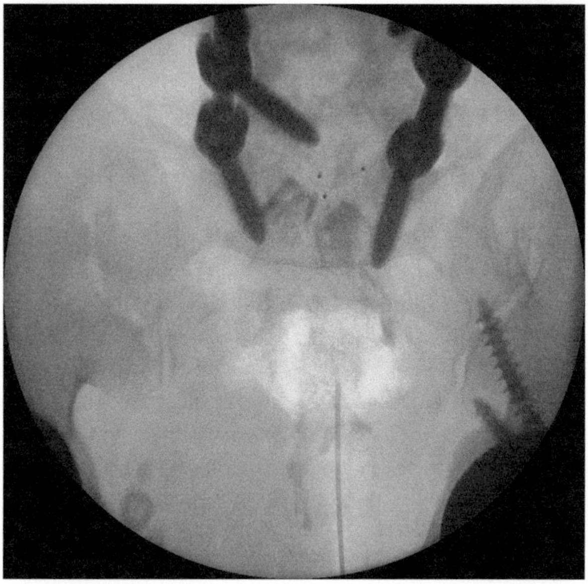

Fig. 10.1 Anteroposterior and lateral fluoroscopic views depicting pelvic structures and lower vertebrae of the lumbar spine. The spinal needle is seen entering at the sacral hiatus and the contrast enhancement of the flow is seen outlining the epidural space. Note globular appearance of the enhancement that follows the epidural fat, which further delineates the flow as epidural

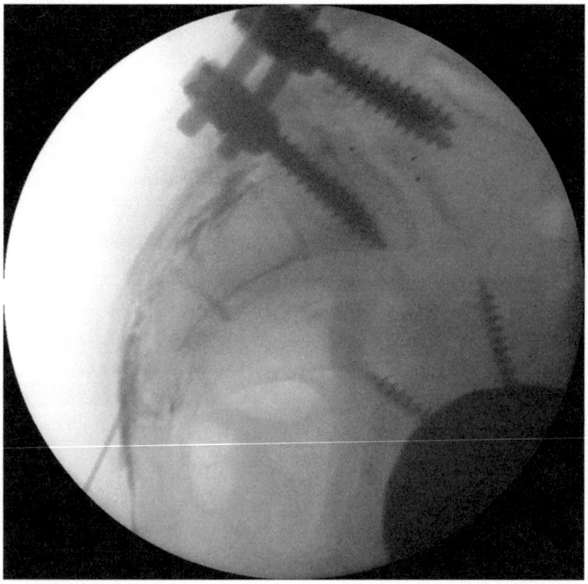

Fig. 10.2 Anteroposterior and lateral fluoroscopic views depicting pelvic structures and lower vertebrae of the lumbar spine. The spinal needle is seen entering at the sacral hiatus and the contrast enhancement of the flow is seen outlining the epidural space. Note globular appearance of the enhancement that follows the epidural fat, which further delineates the flow as epidural

be biased to one side or the other. Because of the occasional and unpredictable presence of a thin connective tissue called plica mediana dorsalis separating left and right dorsal aspects of the epidural space, the medication may flow in a significantly biased amount to one side, limiting the spread to the other.

The transforaminal epidural steroid injection is the most technically demanding of the epidural steroid injection procedures but in many clinical scenarios it is largely considered the most efficacious. In this procedure, a needle is advanced to the intervertebral foramina around the posterolateral margin of the disc (Fig. 10.3). This is the most ventral approach and therefore allows the most amount of medication to be delivered to the intended site [9]. There are several important considerations with this technique. If there is even a partial vascular flow of the medication due to needle placement, then an intravascular injection may occur. This becomes particularly important if the practitioner is using medication that has particulate matter. Occlusion of a radicular artery due to vascular injection of particulate matter may result in ischemia and its potential sequelae, including the potential for paralysis. Therefore, it is important for the physician to confirm the intended flow via live contrast injection that shows appropriate spread of the medication and no vascular uptake. If necessary, the physician should use digital subtraction for added clarity of injection if vascular uptake is at all in question.

Another consideration with the transforaminal approach is the plica mediana dorsalis which may provide a more concentrated unilateral spread of the medication but decreases the potential benefit of diffuse reduction of inflammation at the

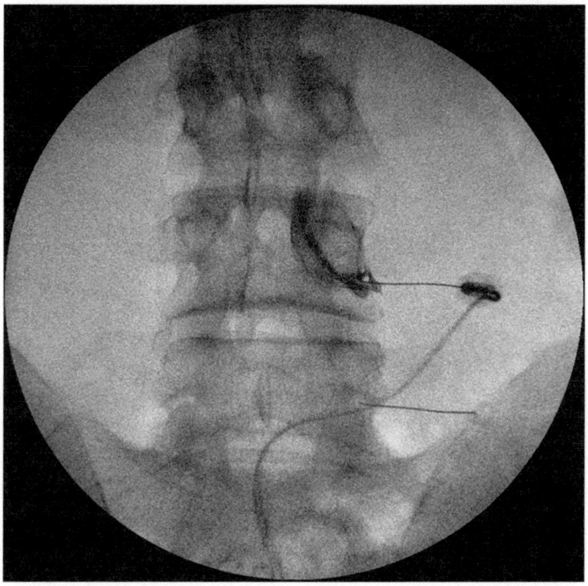

Fig. 10.3 Needle placement for transformational epidural injections at the right L4–L5 and right L5–S1 intervertebral foramina, targeting right L4 and L5 spinal nerves. Epidural contrast flow can be seen at the L4–L5 intervertebral foramen

contralateral side, possibly necessitating the need for a bilateral injection in the case of bilateral symptoms. Ultimately, the primary advantage of the transforaminal approach is a maximum concentrated amount of medication at the site of injection. This is an advantage if the appropriate level is selected for injection, and it also allows the transforaminal approach to be used diagnostically. However, if the symptoms are diffusely spread, or if the appropriate level is not selected, then an alternate mode of injection may be preferred.

When epidural steroid injections are utilized for a lumbosacral radiculopathy, it is important for both the physician and the patient to recognize that even when successful, the injection does not change the anatomy or underlying biomechanics that led to the symptoms in the first place. The symptoms are not "masked" as it is not painkiller that is injected. Rather, the inflammation has been reduced and with the reduction of inflammation, the pain is also reduced. For this reason, it is very important to utilize the time when the patient is feeling better after an injection to focus on stretching and strengthening exercises to address the spinal biomechanics so that the inflammation and pain do not return.

The subject of efficacy for (and against) epidural steroid injections in the literature is a place of active contention [10]. Double-blind placebo-controlled studies have failed to show long-term efficacy of epidural steroid injections for radiculopathies, but prospective and retrospective outcome studies have mostly shown good results. How does one square those two sets of data? The most important point to realize is that double-blind prospective studies that have failed to show therapeutic benefit from epidural steroid injections for radiculopathies have looked at the injection in isolation without the benefit of concomitant structured physical therapy exercises. Of course, in these studies the benefit of the injection has proven to be short lived. By contrast, prospective outcome studies and retrospective studies as well as an overwhelming wealth of empiric clinical data suggest that injections can be very effective when combined with physical therapy exercises [11–14]. What is sorely lacking is a prospective, double-blind placebo-controlled study that incorporates physical therapy following the injection. Further, the study needs to evaluate efficacy in lumbosacral radiculopathies from different causes. Specifically, the efficacy of the injection coupled to physical therapy likely is somewhat different in younger patients with disc herniations versus older patients with multifactorial spinal stenosis [15].

If the pain is persistent despite epidural steroid injections and physical therapy and if that pain is very significant, then surgery is considered. The two primary indications for surgery for a radiculopathy are pain that is not responding to conservative measures and is significant enough to consider surgery and progressive neurologic loss. If a patient is becoming weaker or progressively losing feeling in the leg, then a surgical consult should be sought emergently and surgery should be strongly considered to stop the progressive neurologic loss. Surgery does not always allow patients to regain the neurologic loss, but it should stop the loss from becoming worse.

Surgery to address a radiculopathy generally consists of decompression of the nerve root. If by decompressing the nerve root the spine would potentially become destabilized, then decompression and fusion may be required. Decompression surgeries are naturally less invasive than fusion surgeries and involve less surgical risk, less recovery and rehabilitation time, and less risk of adjacent level disease and therefore the threshold for a patient to undergo decompressive surgery should generally be lower than for fusion surgeries.

References and Suggested Further Reading

1. Tarulli AW, Raynor EM. Lumbosacral radiculopathy. Neurol Clin. 2007;25(2):387–405.
2. Braddom RL, editor. Physical medicine and rehabilitation. Philadelphia, PA: WB Saunders; 1996. p. 844–6.
3. Tarulli AW, Raynor EM. Lumbosacral radiculopathy. Neurol Clin. 2007;25(2):387–405.
4. Borenstein DG, O'Mara JWJR, Boden SD, et al. The value of magnetic resonance imaging of the lumbar spine to predict low back pain in asymptomatic subjects: a seven year follow-up study. J Bone Joint Surg Am. 2001;83-A(9):1306–11.
5. Padua L, Commodari I, Zappia M, Pazzaglia C, Tonali PA. Misdiagnosis of lumbar-sacral radiculopathy: usefulness of combination of EMG and ultrasound. Neurol Sci. 2007;28(3):154–5.
6. Tong HC. Incremental ability of needle electromyography to detect radiculopathy in patients with radiating low back pain using different diagnostic criteria. Arch Phys Med Rehabil. 2012;93(6):990–2.
7. Akuthota V, Nadler SF. Core strengthening. Arch Phys Med Rehabil. 2004;85(3 suppl 1):S86–92.
8. Lutz GE, Vad VB, Wisneski RJ. Fluoroscopic transforaminal lumbar epidural steroids: an outcome study. Arch Phys Med Rehabil. 1998;79(11):1362–6.
9. Derby R, Bogduk N, Kine G. Precision percutaneous blocking procedures for localizing spinal pain. Part 2. The lumbar neuraxial compartment. Pain Digest. 1993;3:175–88.
10. DePalma MJ, Bhargava A, Slipman CW. A critical appraisal of the evidence for selective nerve root injection in the treatment of lumbosacral radiculopathy. Arch Phys Med Rehabil. 2005;86(7):1477–83.
11. Weiner BK, Fraser RD. Foraminal injection for lateral lumbar disc herniation. J Bone Joint Surg Br. 1997;79:804–7.
12. Lutz GE, Vad VB, Wiskenski RJ. Fluoroscopic transforaminal lumbar epidural steroids: an outcome study. Arch Phys Med Rehabil. 1997;79:1362–6.
13. Botwin KP, Gruber RD, Bouchlas CG, et al. Fluoroscopically guided lumbar transforaminal epidural steroid injections in degenerative lumbar stenosis: an outcome study. Am J Phys Med Rehabil. 2002;81:898–905.
14. Vad VB, Bhat AL, Lutz GE, et al. Transforaminal epidural steroid injections in lumbosacral radiculopathy: a prospective randomized study. Spine. 2002;27:11–6.
15. Ng LC, Sell P. Outcomes of a prospective cohort study on peri-radicular infiltration for radicular pain in patients with lumbar disc herniation and spinal stenosis. Eur Spine J. 2004;13:325–9.
16. Gharibo CG, Varlotta GP, Rhame EE, Liu EC, Bendo JA, Perloff MD. Interlaminar versus transforaminal epidural steroids for the treatment of subacute lumbar radicular pain: a randomized, blinded, prospective outcome study. Pain Physician. 2011;14(6):499–511.

Chapter 11
Piriformis Syndrome

The function of the piriformis muscle is to externally rotate the hip when the hip is in extension and to abduct the hip when it is in flexion. In approximately 20 % of the population, the piriformis muscle belly is split and one or more parts of the sciatic nerve passes through the piriformis muscle [1]. Typically, when it passes through, it is the peroneal portion of the sciatic nerve that pierces the piriformis muscle. The sciatic nerve itself, as a single nerve, is the largest in the human body. Historically, piriformis syndrome has been an overused diagnosis as it has been conflated with a lumbosacral radiculopathy which epidemiologically is much more common. Because the L5, S1, and S2 nerve roots innervate the piriformis muscle, the piriformis muscle is often tight and in spasm in the presence of a lumbosacral radiculopathy. Further, because the L5 and S1 nerve roots are so commonly inflamed, and because these spinal nerves are the primary feeders of the sciatic nerve, the diagnosis of piriformis syndrome or "sciatica" is often given when in fact the L5 and/or S1 nerve roots are the actual cause. In fact, true piriformis syndrome involves irritation or inflammation of the piriformis muscle that may result in compression or inflammation of the sciatic nerve.

Consider the following patient: Samantha is a 34-year-old attorney who is an avid early morning runner. While training for a marathon, she developed right buttock pain radiating into her right posterior thigh. The pain is worse with running and better when she lies down. Sitting does not make the pain worse although sometimes she has increased pain with transitioning from sit to stand after she has been sitting for a while. She has some numbness in the right lateral lower leg after a long run. On exam, she has a negative straight leg raise. Her piriformis muscle is very tender and pressure reproduces sciatic symptoms into the right thigh. MRI of her lumbar spine is normal and electrodiagnostic tests are within normal limits.

Most spine specialists would agree that Samantha is likely suffering from piriformis syndrome. Piriformis syndrome is often suspected when a patient presents with Samantha's symptoms and then on exam she is found to have significant tenderness in the piriformis muscle. However, if all the examining physicians knew Samantha's history and the fact that her piriformis muscle was very tender and that palpation

G. Cooper, *Non-Operative Treatment of the Lumbar Spine*,
DOI 10.1007/978-3-319-21443-6_11

reproduced her symptoms, then a diagnosis of piriformis syndrome would *still* be premature and likely incorrect. An L5–S1 radiculopathy would present in the same way and the piriformis muscle would likely be just as tender because it may spasm in response to the nerve root inflammation. However, the fact that the dural root tension sign is negative (straight leg raise) is Samantha's case further supports the diagnosis of piriformis syndrome. Still, a diagnosis at that point of the work-up would be premature. For Samantha, it is the fact that she has all of the above features *and* the fact that her lumbosacral MRI is normal *and* that the electrodiagnostic studies were normal that suggest the diagnosis piriformis syndrome.

If Samantha had a positive straight leg raise *or* an L5–S1 disc herniation *or* electrodiagnostic studies revealing an L5 and S1 radiculopathy, then that would have been the most likely diagnosis. Even with all of the above data points, it is still not definitive that Samantha has piriformis syndrome but it certainly appears that she does. In the end, piriformis syndrome remains a clinical diagnosis without a gold standard test.

When a lumbosacral radiculopathy is excluded and piriformis syndrome is the presumptive diagnosis, treatment typically begins with physical therapy. The physical therapy will focus on stretching the piriformis muscle as well as the other hip muscles. Passive modalities such as ultrasound and soft tissue mobilization are often used to stretch the hip joint capsule as well as the involved and surrounding muscles. Lumbar stabilization exercises are often incorporated into the physical therapy program. If an activity such as running is felt to have been contributing to the development of the piriformis syndrome, then it is important to evaluate the gait and address any suboptimal mechanics. In addition, the mechanics of the feet should be evaluated in an instance such as running contributing to piriformis syndrome and orthotics may be considered.

If the symptoms do not respond to physical therapy and home exercises, or if the symptoms are too severe to allow the patient to participate with the exercise regimen, then a trigger point into the piriformis muscle is often used. Ideally, ultrasound guidance is used for the injection in order to ensure proper localization of the needle into the belly of the piriformis muscle as well as to ensure avoidance of any vascular structures and also to avoid direct injection into the sciatic nerve [2]. The trigger point injection for piriformis syndrome often uses a small dose of steroid in addition to lidocaine or bupivacaine.

If piriformis syndrome is not responding to physical therapy and a trigger point injection with steroid then some doctors feel botulinum toxin injection may be helpful [3, 4]. The goal of using botulinum toxin (e.g., Botox) is to relax the muscle and facilitate further physical therapy. The main risk of botulinum toxin injection in this instance is to paralyze the muscle too much in which case the gait may be thrown off further and this may potentially lead to other musculoskeletal problems.

As a last resort, surgical release of the piriformis muscle in which the piriformis tendon is loosened may be considered if symptoms are ongoing and debilitating and symptoms have not improved with aggressive conservative care. Surgical release for piriformis syndrome should be rare as conservative care is generally effective.

References and Suggested Further Reading

1. Jankiewicz JJ, Hennrikus WL, Houkom JA. The appearance of the piriformis muscle syndrome in computed tomography and magnetic resonance imaging. A case report and review of the literature. Clin Orthop. 1991;262:205–9.
2. Blunk JA, Nowotny M, Scharf J, Benrath J. MRI verification of ultrasound-guided infiltrations of local anesthetics into the piriformis muscle. Pain Med. 2013;14(10):1593–9.
3. Fishman LM, Konnoth C, Rozner B. Botulinum neurotoxin type B and physical therapy in the treatment of piriformis syndrome: a dose finding study. Am J Phys Med Rehabil. 2004;83(1):42–50. quiz 51-53.
4. Fishman LM, Anderson C, Rosner B. BOTOX and physical therapy in the treatment of piriformis syndrome. Am J Phys Med Rehabil. 2002;81(12):936–42.
5. Syasyon SC, Ducey JP, Maybrey JB, et al. Sciatic entrapment neuropathy associated with an anomalous piriformis muscle. Pain. 1994;59(1):149–52.
6. Dezawa A, Kusano S, Miki H. Arthroscopic release of the piriformis muscle under local anesthesia for piriformis syndrome. Arthroscopy. 2003;19(5):554–7.
7. Rossi P, Cardinali P, Serrao M, et al. Magnetic resonance imaging findings in piriformis syndrome: a case report. Arch Phys Med Rehabil. 2001;82(4):519–21.
8. Vandertop WP, Bosma NJ. The piriformis syndrome. A case report. J Bone Joint Surg Am. 1991;73(7):1095–7.

Chapter 12
Spinal Stenosis

The words spinal stenosis have a Greek origin. The word "stenosis" means "choking." Spinal, of course, means spine. So spinal stenosis is a choking (or narrowing) of the spine canal. While anything that narrows the spinal canal (e.g., a disc herniation) will create stenosis, conventionally when "spinal stenosis" is used as a diagnosis, it refers to a predominance of the stenosis originating from the posterior elements (e.g., facet joint arthropathy, buckled ligamentum flavum) although there is often an element of disc herniation contributing to the stenosis.

The anatomic finding of some degree of spinal stenosis is "part of aging" in the sense that after the age of 65, just about everyone is going to have some degree of spinal stenosis on MRI [1, 2]. Of course, not everyone over the age of 65 has symptoms from their spinal stenosis. Indeed, most people do not. Even in patients with spinal stenosis and symptoms, there are typically other levels within that patient's spine that reveal some amount of stenosis without symptomatology.

When spinal stenosis does cause symptoms, the symptoms do not generally occur because of a true compression of the spinal nerves but rather the reduced space in the spinal canal creates a greater propensity for the patient to develop inflammation around the nerve roots as a result of the stenosis and this leads to symptoms. In rare cases the nerves may become truly mechanically compressed in which case the symptoms are generally severe and progressive.

Common symptoms of spinal stenosis include lower back pain radiating into the legs. The symptoms are generally worse with standing and walking and relieved with sitting or bending forward. Other symptoms may include numbness and tingling in the legs. Patients may also complain of a lack of feeling steady on their feet. A common sign is something called the shopping cart sign. In this sign, a patient describes being unable to walk more than 5 min but then says that they can walk for a half hour with ease in the shopping center when they are bent over on the shopping cart. While it is often assumed by the patient that this is because they are leaning their weight onto the cart, it is in fact due to the fact that they are flexed forward while leaning on the shopping cart, which alleviates the pressure from their spinal nerves.

G. Cooper, *Non-Operative Treatment of the Lumbar Spine*,
DOI 10.1007/978-3-319-21443-6_12

Consider the following patient. Charles is a 78-year-old male with a 5-year history of progressively worsening lower back pain radiating into the bilateral posterior and lateral thighs and lower legs. His legs feel heavy when he walks. He can walk about 10 min before he has to sit down. As soon as he sits down, the pain goes away. On physical examination, he has 4+/5 bilateral hip abductor strength and decreased sensation to light touch in the bilateral soles of the feet but is otherwise neurologically intact. He has pain and restricted movement with trunk extension and bilateral oblique extension.

Most spine specialists would agree that Charles probably has spinal stenosis causing bilateral lumbosacral radiculopathies. MRI of the lumbosacral spine would likely reveal moderate multilevel spinal stenosis. If vascular claudication is suspected then Dopplers may be obtained. An inexpensive way to differentiate vascular claudication from spinal stenosis symptoms is to have a patient walk and also use an exercise bicycle. If the patient has spinal stenosis causing his symptoms, then he should have the leg symptoms while walking but he should not have the leg symptoms when using a bicycle. This is because his is in a trunk flexed position while on the bicycle which takes the pressure off his nerves. If on the other hand the symptoms are due to vascular causes, then the symptoms should limit his ability to walk as well as to ride a bicycle. This is because in vascular claudication it is the demand for oxygen that causes the symptoms in the legs and so walking and bicycling both create that demand and the position of the patient's trunk is immaterial.

Initial treatment for lumbar spinal stenosis typically involves physical therapy that focuses on lumbar stabilization and hip strengthening exercises and hip flexor and knee extensor stretching. Passive modalities are often used as well to reduce overlying myofascial pain and adhesions. If symptoms are not improving with physical therapy, or if the symptoms make it difficult to participate with physical therapy, then an epidural steroid injection may be helpful. It should be emphasized that an epidural steroid injection does not "fix" the underlying stenosis. An epidural steroid injection is also not a "Band-Aid" in that it is not a painkiller. Rather, an epidural steroid injection helps reduce the swelling and inflammation from around an inflamed nerve root. When an epidural steroid injection is able to reduce this swelling and remove the symptoms, it should be coupled to physical therapy exercises in order to maximize the biomechanics and help reduce the pressure from the spinal canal so that ideally the symptoms do not recur [4].

Epidural steroid injections are more effective for foraminal stenosis than for central stenosis. For a more complete discussion of epidural steroid injections, see the previous chapters on lumbosacral radiculopathy and discogenic lower back pain. For multiple pathologies, long-term outcomes rest more in participation and compliance with therapeutic exercise regimens and postural and ergonomic adjustments than with lone injections. However, this is particularly true when considering spinal stenosis. Studies have repeatedly shown that epidural steroid injections for spinal stenosis offer good short-term relief but inconsistent long-term outcomes after 6 months or a year [5, 6]. It is also important to note that studies have also shown poor compliance with therapeutic exercises after 6 months to a year. The sum results of these datum is the importance that the physician articulates the necessity of learning and participating in a consistent therapeutic exercise program as well as improved ergonomic and postural habits and possibly activity modification in order to achieve the desired long-term results.

Inherent to symptomatic spinal stenosis is the potential for limited mobility and this can have negative psychological ramifications. It is important that physicians be aware of this potential and help patients to identify this in themselves. Sometimes simply acknowledging the legitimacy of the stress helps patients to cope with it or opens an avenue for them to find help in developing coping strategies.

When conservative care has not been helpful and the pain is significant and not controlled with oral pain medications, then another potential therapeutic intervention is a spinal cord stimulator. A spinal cord stimulator is a procedure that does not fix the spinal stenosis but it is designed to distract and ideally eliminate the patient's pain. A spinal cord stimulator has two steps to its implementation. The first step is a spinal cord stimulator trial. This is a percutaneous procedure in which a catheter is used to introduce wires that will rest on the appropriate levels of the dorsal columns of the spinal cord. Those wires are connected to a small computer-controlled battery pack that the patient carries around for a week. This battery pack usually will contain a certain degree of patient control. The idea is that the patient can increase or decrease the amount of stimulation to his spinal cord. The ultimate goal is for the patient to feel the sensation from the stimulation instead of the pain. Then ultimately, the brain may attenuate to the buzzing or other sensation from the stimulation and simply not feel the pain. Often a patient will be instructed to use it for a few hours several times per day. The regimen of course depends on the patient's particular clinical scenario.

If the patient receives good pain relief that is meaningful in the context of the patient's activities of daily living from the spinal cord stimulator trial, then the stimulator may be surgically implanted. Careful consideration should be taken when selecting the appropriate stimulator. If the spinal cord is implanted, then the patient will receive a wireless remote to be able to control the intensity and duration of the pulse strength. With recent advances in technology, the stimulators have been improving and each has its own relative advantages and disadvantages. For example, for those with a more active lifestyle, it is important to select a stimulator that can adapt to the changes of rapid flexion and extension of the spine as well as changes in horizontal and vertical positions of the body by regulating the pulse strength. This allows for adequate pain control without unwanted spikes in pulse that can otherwise be quite uncomfortable.

Another consideration for spinal cord stimulator selection is the battery in terms of both its life and the process for recharging it. Most spinal cord stimulators have batteries that will last for several years and can be easily recharged. Another consideration is a potential for the patient to need magnetic resonance imaging (MRI) in the future. Most implantable devices are not compatible with MRI although some devices make it possible to perform some limited MRI in other parts of the body.

It is important to realize that if a spinal cord stimulator is effective at controlling a patient's pain, the underlying condition has not actually been fixed. Therefore, it is important to monitor a patient's potential progression of neurologic deficits.

Surgery for lumbar stenosis is indicated when there is significant pain that is affecting quality of life and not getting better with conservative care or when there is progressive neurologic loss. The two basic types of surgery involve a laminectomy or laminectomy with fusion surgery. X-STOP is another surgery for lumbar stenosis in which a device is inserted between the spinous processes to help flex and open the spinal canal. MILD is another minimally invasive surgical procedure in which the posterior elements of the spinal canal are targeted in order to decompress the spine. Surgery in patients with spinal stenosis is generally very effective at reducing or eliminating the leg pain and preventing the progression of neurologic symptoms but is generally less effective in addressing the symptom of lower back pain and is variable in terms of reversing neurologic symptoms [7].

An alternative to surgery or a treatment path if surgery is ineffective or inadequate at controlling a patient's pain is an intrathecal pump that delivers medication directly to the subarachnoid space. An intrathecal pump provides a baseline level of medication to provide baseline pain control in addition to the option of delivering increased medication in the event of breakthrough pain. Restrictions within the pump are created in order to help avoid overdose. By delivering the medication directly to the intrathecal space, a much more concentrated dose of medication may be used with less chance of significant side effects. Common medications used in an intrathecal pump include opioids, adrenergic agonists, local anesthetics, GABA-B receptor agonists, ziconotide, and *N*-methyl-D-aspartate receptor agonists as well as a variety of other medications. An intrathecal pump goes through a similar process as a spinal cord stimulator with an initial trial and, if successful in decreasing the pain without unwanted significant side effects, then a surgically implanted intrathecal pump may be placed. An intrathecal pump requires more ongoing management than a spinal cord stimulator. In addition to having to consider the battery life, the reservoir of medication must be refilled on a regular basis.

References and Suggested Further Reading

1. Borenstein DG, O'Mara JWJR, Boden SD, et al. The value of magnetic resonance imaging of the lumbar spine to predict low back pain in asymptomatic subjects: a seven year follow-up study. J Bone Joint Surg Am. 2001;83-A(9):1306–11.
2. Greenberg JO, Schnell RG. Magnetic resonance imaging of the lumbar spine in asymptomatic adults. Cooperative study – American Society of Neuroimaging. J Neuroimaging. 1991;1(1):2–7.
3. Simotas AC, Dorey FJ, Hansraj KK, Cammisa Jr F. Nonoperative treatment for lumbar spinal stenosis. Clinical and outcome results and a 3-year survivorship analysis. Spine (Phila Pa 1976). 2000;25(2):197–203. discussions 203–4.
4. Abdi S, Datta S, Trescot AM, Schultz DM, Adlaka R, Atluri SL, Smith HS, Manchikanti L. Epidural steroids in the management of chronic spinal pain: a systematic review. Pain Physician. 2007;10(1):185–212.
5. Manchikanti L, Buenaventura RM, Manchikanti KN, Ruan X, Gupta S, Smith HS, Christo PJ, Ward SP. Effectiveness of therapeutic lumbar transforaminal epidural steroid injections in managing lumbar spinal pain. Pain Physician. 2012;15(3):E199–245.

6. Kreiner DS, Shaffer WO, Baisden JL, Gilbert TJ, Summers JT, Toton JF, et al. An evidence-based clinical guideline for the diagnosis and treatment of degenerative lumbar spinal stenosis (update). Spine J. 2013;13(7):734–43.
7. NASS Evidence-Based Clinical Guidelines Committee. Diagnosis and treatment of degenerative lumbar spinal stenosis (2011 Revised). Burr Ridge: North American Spine Society; 2011. NASS evidence-based clinical guidelines for multidisciplinary spine care.
8. Cinotti G, De Santis P, Nofroni I, et al. Stenosis of the intervertebral foramen. Anatomic study on predisposing factors. Spine. 2002;27:223–9.
9. Iguchi T, Kurihara A, Nakayama J, et al. Minimum 10-yearoutcome of decompressive laminectomy for degenerative lumbar spinal stenosis. Spine. 2000;25:1754–9.
10. Hansray KKH, Cammisa FP, O'Leary PF, et al. Decompressive surgery for typical lumbar spinal stenosis. Clin Ortop. 2001;384:11–7.

Chapter 13
Compression Fractures

Compression fractures may occur in the vertebrae and cause lower back pain. They most commonly occur in patients with osteoporosis. Osteoporosis weakens the bone leading that bone vulnerable to fracture from everyday activities of daily living (e.g., lifting, twisting, coughing) that under normal circumstances would not cause a fracture. Tumors originating from within the spine, or metastases to the spine, may also weaken the bone and result in compression fractures. Significant trauma of course can also result in compression fractures in the spine.

An important fact about compression fractures in the spine is that they can be asymptomatic. Indeed, sometimes, the patient has a compression fracture and no recollection of any back pain. Consider that it has been estimated that a quarter of postmenopausal females have had at least one vertebral compression fracture. Sometimes a patient may remember an episode of lower back pain but that pain subsequently resolved. When lower back pain occurs and a compression fracture is found on an imaging test, it is important to take the fracture seriously, consider why it is there, and consider that it is a potential source of the lower back pain, but it is also important to recognize that the pain may be originating from another source within the spine and that the compression fracture may be incidental to the pain.

Consider the following patient. Eleanor is an 82-year-old female who presents with 2 weeks of severe lower back pain. She has a history of hypertension and osteoporosis but was otherwise doing okay until she lifted her granddaughter 2 weeks ago and immediately felt a sharp pain in the upper part of her lower back. The pain has been so intense that she has been mostly bedbound for the last 2 weeks. She went to her primary care doctor who ordered an X-ray that revealed an L1 compression fracture, multilevel facet joint arthropathy, and degenerative disc disease. On physical examination she is neurologically intact and has severe point tenderness over the anatomic location consistent with her L1 spinal segment. Trunk movement of any kind while standing intensifies the pain.

Most spine specialists would agree that Eleanor is suffering from an acute L1 compression fracture. An MRI is often obtained in order to evaluate the extent of the fracture as well as to evaluate the nerves. A CT may be obtained if there is not a

G. Cooper, *Non-Operative Treatment of the Lumbar Spine*,
DOI 10.1007/978-3-319-21443-6_13

concern for neurologic damage and if an invasive procedure such as kyphoplasty of vertebroplasty to address the pain is being considered. When a compression fracture is identified, it is important to treat the pain from the fracture as well as to make sure that the underlying cause of the fracture (e.g., osteoporosis in Eleanor's case) is being optimally managed. If a compression fracture is found in an older patient who has not had a recent DEXA scan then it is important to obtain one. If a compression fracture is found in a younger patient with no other obvious cause for the fracture (e.g., tumor), then a DEXA scan should be included as part of the work-up as to why the fracture occurred.

Initial treatment of a compression fracture is nonsurgical and involves relative rest and pain medications. Physical therapy is often started in order to maximize the movement that can be tolerated. Especially in patients with underlying osteoporosis, bed rest can lead to worsening of that osteoporosis as well as put the patient at risk for a thromboembolic event so mobilization is important. Physical therapy will often incorporate heat and gentle massage for pain relief. The exercises in physical therapy should target flexibility and lumbar stabilization exercises with an extension bias used for the exercises [1, 2]. In years past, extension bracing was commonly used, but this has become controversial because of the extra stress that bracing places on the posterior elements of the spine. As such, it is no longer considered the standard of care but can be used in select cases.

Most cases of compression fractures will improve with noninterventional care. However, if the pain is intolerable or does not improve over 6–8 weeks, then vertebroplasty and kyphoplasty are two interventional treatments that may be considered for painful compression fractures [3]. In both of these procedures, a needle or surgical device is inserted into the compression fracture. In vertebroplasty, cement is injected under high pressure to stabilize the fracture. The advantage of vertebroplasty is that it is relatively quicker than kyphoplasty. The disadvantage is that high pressure is used and this can lead to complications such as cement emboli. Additionally, as opposed to kyphoplasty, the height of the bone is not restored. In kyphoplasty, surgical instrumentation is placed into the fracture and a balloon is inflated that creates a vacuum into which cement is injected. The two advantages of kyphoplasty are that the procedure is done under relatively low pressure, minimizing cement emboli, and also height is restored to the fractured vertebral body. Both vertebroplasty and kyphoplasty are effective at quickly reducing the pain from an osteoporotic compression fracture; however, both suffer from the criticism that they may potentially increase the risk of adjacent-level compression fractures [4]. This remains a point of ongoing research and some contention. In the meantime, vertebroplasty and kyphoplasty are appropriate surgical options for patients with severe pain who are not responding to more conservative measures.

In patients with chronic pain and radiographic evidence of an old compression fracture, it is critical to realize that the compression fracture may not be the source of pain. In addition to the usual more common causes of lower back pain (e.g., discogenic pain), it has been found that the incidence of facet joint pain may increase in the presence of osteoporotic compression fractures [5]. This is believed to be because the biomechanical stress that used to pass through the vertebral body is now instead translated disproportionally through the facet joints. Therefore, medial branch blocks of the facet joints should be strongly considered in patients with chronic back pain even when an osteoporotic compression fracture is identified and suspected as being the source of the pain. Naturally, an additional point to consider is that there may be, and often is, more than one pain generator and since a pain generator such as a facet joint is ultimately treatable with radiofrequency rhizotomy, it is worth knowing if that is a significant portion of the pain as it can be more readily eliminated using conservative options than can chronic pain from an osteoporotic compression fracture.

In a 2009 placebo-controlled study examining the efficacy of vertebroplasty, it was found that vertebroplasty did not reveal a statistically significant difference in the main outcome of pain when compared with sham procedure [6]. However, the sham procedure involved anesthetizing the injection site as well as the subcutaneous tissues and the periosteum overlying the pedicle through which the needle for the vertebroplasty would be inserted. This location also had the effect of anesthetizing the medial branch of the facet joint. It has been postulated that although the study aimed to look solely at the efficacy of vertebroplasty to reduce the patient's pain, some specialists argued that it showed support for the biomechanical model in which the facet joints mediate a significant portion of the pain following compression fracture as previous studies have indicated that simply anesthetizing the medial branch has the effect of reducing pain in facet joint mediated lower back pain.

References and Suggested Further Reading

1. Freedman BA, Potter BK, Nesti LJ, et al. Osteoporosis and vertebral compression fractures-continued missed opportunities. Spine J. 2008;8:756.
2. Prather H, Watson JO, Gilula LA. Nonoperative management of osteoporotic vertebral compression fractures. Injury. 2007;38 Suppl 3:S40–8.
3. Karlsson MK, Hasserius R, Gerdhem P, et al. Vertebroplasty and kyphoplasty: new treatment strategies for fractures in the osteoporotic spine. Acta Orthop. 2005;76(5):620–7.
4. Movrin I, Vengust R, Komadina R. Adjacent vertebral fractures after percutaneous vertebral augmentation of osteoporotic vertebral compression fracture: a comparison of balloon kyphoplasty and vertebroplasty. Arch Orthop Trauma Surg. 2010;130(9):1157–66. doi:10.1007/s00402-010-1106-3. Epub 2010 May 7.
5. Park KD MD, Jee H PhD, Nam HS MD, Cho SK MD, Kim HS MD, Park Y MD, Lim OK MD. Effect of medial branch block in chronic facet joint pain for osteoporotic compression fracture: one year retrospective study. Ann Rehabil Med. 2013;37(2):191–201.
6. Buchbinder R, Osborne RH, Ebeling PR, Wark JD, Mitchell P, Wriedt C, Graves S, Staples MP, Murphy B. A randomized trial of vertebroplasty for painful osteoporotic vertebral fractures. N Engl J Med. 2009;361(6):557–68. doi:10.1056/NEJMoa0900429.
7. Lieberman IH, Dudeney S, Reinhardt MK, et al. Initial outcome and efficacy of 'kyphoplasty' in the treatment of painful osteoporotic vertebral compression fractures. Spine. 2001;26:1631–8.
8. Silverman SL. The clinical consequences of vertebral compression fracture. Bone. 1992;13 Suppl 2:S27–31.
9. Berlemann U, Ferguson SJ, Nolte LP, et al. Adjacent vertebral failure after vertebroplasty. A biomechanical investigation. J Bone Joint Surg Br. 2002;84:748–52.

Chapter 14
Epidural Steroid Injections: Dispelling Common Myths

Perhaps there is no source of confusion, contention, obfuscation, and general misunderstandings primarily among patients but also doctors as there is in regard to epidural steroid injections. This chapter is devoted to trying to dispel some of the more common myths.

Epidural steroid injections do not correct any anatomical or biomechanical problems leading to a radiculopathy. Epidural steroid injections, however, do not mask pain or "put a Band-Aid" on the problem. Epidural steroid injections work by serving to reduce the swelling and inflammation around an inflamed nerve root. When used in isolation, epidural steroid injections have not been shown to provide good, consistent long-term relief. When used as a tool to enable patients to participate with structured therapeutic exercises, they have been shown to have good efficacy. However, in the end the data as it stands is mixed and a large part of the resulting confusion lies in the fact that prospective, double-blind placebo-controlled studies in an effort to evaluate *only* the injection have not included structured physical therapy as part of the study design. As a result, in many of these studies only short-term benefit is seen from the injection. Short-term benefit should be the norm to be expected from most steroid injections for a variety of musculoskeletal pathologies as they address inflammation, not biomechanics. Prospective cohort outcome studies and retrospective studies, by contrast, follow patients through a normal treatment paradigm which does *or at least should* include therapeutic exercises, and these studies have tended to show good longer-term efficacy for epidural steroid injections [1–3]. Of course, it should be emphasized and reemphasized that these studies do not show good long-term effect of the injection alone but rather as it is used as part of a more comprehensive treatment paradigm. What is clearly needed are double-blind placebo-controlled studies that incorporate physical therapy as well as the injection procedures and that also look at this paradigm as it relates to patients with herniated discs causing radiculopathy as well as multifactorial spinal stenosis causing radiculopathy.

The number and frequency of epidural steroid injections remains a topic that lacks data and consensus in equal parts. Many doctors tell each other and their

G. Cooper, *Non-Operative Treatment of the Lumbar Spine*,
DOI 10.1007/978-3-319-21443-6_14

patients that there should be a limit of three epidural steroid injections in a six-month time frame or sometimes even in a year. However, this is based in dogma, not research. Three injections is a fine number, but why not four or seven or two or even one? As there is no data, there really is no good answer. What is established is that steroid injections may locally degrade cartilage and will weaken tendons and so are and should be used sparingly in joint and tendon injections. There is some systemic absorption of the medication and systemic steroids are known to have many different and serious side effects. The amount of systemic absorption is small but there is at least some suggestion that it may increase fracture risk in elderly patients (see below) and so the potential for problems from systemic absorption should not be completely discounted. However, with regard to the epidural space, it is not known whether there is a local risk of repeated injections. No local risk from repeated epidural steroid injections (other than the risk of any singular injection of infection, bleeding, nerve trauma, and infarction which will be discussed below) has been effectively documented. Some spine surgeons feel that repeated epidural steroid injections performed over the course of years and decades may predispose to an increased complication of dural tearing during a potential spine surgery. However, this conjecture has not been scientifically validated, and the same spine surgeons tend to report that even if that were the case it would not necessarily be a reason to not perform the injections if they are helpful. Insurance companies tend to restrict the number of epidural steroid injections a patient may receive in a year, and this sometimes plays a practical role in decision-making depending on the specific circumstance. However, if the decision of how many injections to perform is based on insurance rather than medical science, this should be effectively communicated to the patient. Insurance denial or restriction does not equate to sound medicine – in this case it merely serves to help perpetuate the dogma.

A 2013 large retrospective analysis revealed evidence that epidural steroid injections in an elderly population increased the risk of fractures by as much as 21 % [4]. The study was retrospective in nature, but it certainly raises concern and should be considered when outlining a treatment strategy on a case-by-case basis. Aside from the retrospective nature of the study, one of the opposing viewpoints in relation to potential future fracture is that to the extent that an epidural steroid injection allows a patient to participate in weight-bearing exercise and increase mobility, and to the extent that it is used in this mode, it may serve to prevent subsequent fracture risk. This too will ideally be sorted through future research.

Epidural steroid injections are generally considered safe. Infection and bleeding are risks of any procedure, but these risks are minimal with infections occurring generally at a rate of 0.1–0.01 % of injections. In a reported review in 2014 of over 14,960 lumbosacral epidural steroid injections, there were no reported cases of infection, neurologic deficit, or hemorrhage [5]. Still, infection and bleeding must always be considered.

Bleeding in the context of an epidural approach has a different consideration than other injection procedures. A hematoma occurring within the epidural space is confined and limited in expansion by the spinal canal and thus may compress the spinal cord or spinal nerves. Patients with coagulopathies need special consideration and at times may require premedication. Patients on blood thinners also require special consideration and patients may need to stop their blood thinners prior to their epidural steroid injection depending on the particular blood thinner and clinical scenario. Platelet inhibiting medications are surrounded by controversy in the context of spinal procedures and epidurals in particular with some physicians and spine organizations arguing that the relative risk of a hematoma is lower than the potential risk of stopping the medication. This remains an area of ongoing research, debate, and scrutiny.

Dural puncture is a complication of an epidural in which the needle tip punctures the dura. This has been reported overall in approximately 0.5 % of epidurals. In the same previously mentioned recent study of 14,960 lumbosacral epidural steroid injections, dural puncture was reported at a rate of 0.3 % in interlaminar lumbar epidural steroid injections and <0.1 % of transforaminal epidurals steroid injections. A dural puncture may result in severe positional headaches in which the patient has pain when vertical such as sitting or standing and no pain while horizontal such as lying down. The headache usually begins within 12–24 h after the epidural injection. The majority of these headaches resolve spontaneously within 48 h. If the headache does not improve or if the pain is severe then a blood patch may be used in which blood is drawn from the patient and then injected into the epidural space around the suspected leak in order to help with closure.

Nerve damage from direct trauma from the needle may occur but is exceedingly rare. Fluoroscopically guided epidural steroid injections done under anesthesia may suffer a slight increased complication rate as compared with fluoroscopically guided epidural steroid injections done without anesthesia because the patient is not awake and cannot report pain from the needle as it approaches the nerve, which cannot be seen during needle manipulation under fluoroscopy.

References and Suggested Further Reading

1. Lutz GE, Vad VB, Wiskenski RJ. Fluoroscopic transforaminal lumbar epidural steroids: an outcome study. Arch Phys Med Rehabil. 1997;79:1362–6.
2. Botwin KP, Gruber RD, Bouchlas CG, et al. Fluoroscopically guided lumbar transformational epidural steroid injections in degenerative lumbar stenosis: an outcome study. Am J Phys Med Rehabil. 2002;81:898–905.
3. Vad VB, Bhat AL, Lutz GE, et al. Transforaminal epidural steroid injections in lumbosacral radiculopathy: a prospective randomized study. Spine. 2002;27:11–6.
4. Mandel S, Schilling J, Peterson E, Sudhaker Rao D, Sanders W. A retrospective analysis of vertebral body fractures following epidural steroid injections. J Bone Joint Surg Am. 2013;95(11):961–4.
5. El-Yahchouchi CA, Plastaras CT, Maus TP, Carr CM, McCormick Z, Geske JR, Smuck M, Pingree MJ, Kennedy DJ. Complication rates of transforaminal and interlaminar epidural steroid injections: a multi-institutional study presented at ISIS 2014, winner of Best Abstract Presentation. 2014.

6. Slipman CW, Derby R, Simeone FA, Mayer TG. Interventional spine an algorithmic approach. Philadelphia: Saunders; 2008.
7. McCahon RA, Ravenscroft A, Hodgkinson V, Evley R, Hardman J. A pilot study of the dose-response of caudal methylprednisolone with levobupivacaine in chronic lower back pain. Anaesthesia. 2011;66(7):595–603.
8. Rhee JM, Schaufele M, Abdu WA. Radiculopathy and the herniated lumbar disc. Controversies regarding pathophysiology and management. J Bone Joint Surg Am. 2006;88(9):2070–80.

Chapter 15
Red Flag Signs and Symptoms

Red flag signs and symptoms in the context of lower back pain are signs and symptoms that should prompt further investigation.

Red flag signs and symptoms and what they may indicate include the following:

Fever—risk of infection.
Chills—risk of infection
Recent unexplained weight loss—potential for malignancy
Saddle anesthesia—concern for cauda equina syndrome
Urinary or bowel incontinence—concern for cauda equina syndrome or spinal cord lesion
Progressive weakness or numbness—concern for nerve damage

Any history of cancer, IV drug abuse, HIV, prolonged use of corticosteroids, or other causes of immunosuppression should prompt concern for infection or malignancy and warrant further study depending on the clinical scenario.

History of recent travel to a location with a high incidence of tuberculosis should prompt consideration of tuberculosis in the spine (Pott disease).

Pain that is severe at nighttime and better with activity and during the day may prompt concern for a malignancy depending on the clinical scenario.

Axial lower back and buttock pain in a young male that is much worse in the morning and includes excessive stiffness that can last for over an hour in the morning should prompt concern for ankylosing spondylitis.

G. Cooper, *Non-Operative Treatment of the Lumbar Spine*,
DOI 10.1007/978-3-319-21443-6_15

Chapter 16
Exercises for Lower Back Pain

Exercise is very important for good spine health. Exercise helps spinal health in a number of ways. Exercise to achieve and maintain a healthy weight is important because excess weight places additional unhealthy stresses on the spine. Cardiovascular exercise in general is helpful because good overall health and proper blood flow throughout the body and to the spine aid in achieving spinal health. Weight-bearing exercise is important to help with maintaining good bone density. The most important exercises for spinal health are exercises that target the muscles that directly relieve the pressure from the spine. This chapter focuses on these exercises, but it is important to emphasize to patients that these exercises belong as part of an overall healthy lifestyle and as part of that a broader exercise program.

The specific exercise program designed for a patient's lower back pain will depend on the nature of that patient's lower back pain. When a patient's pain is flexion based (e.g., sitting increases the pain) and believed to be discogenic in origin, then the prescribed exercises will have an extension bias. Reciprocally, when a patient's pain is extension based (e.g., standing increases the pain) then the prescribed exercises have a flexion bias. When pain is neither flexion nor extension based or when both types of positions produce back pain, then the prescribed exercises occur in a neutral spine position.

Every patient needs to be individually evaluated for muscle weaknesses and imbalances. Of course, there are some general principles. The hallmark of many lower back exercise programs includes lumbar stabilization exercises and hip flexor stretching. Two common lumbar stabilization exercises include posterior pelvic tilts and planks.

In a posterior pelvic tilt, the patient lies supine and pushes her belly button into the ground so that the arch of the back disappears (Fig. 16.1). If this becomes easy, heeltaps can be added to the posterior pelvic tilt as long as the pelvic tilt posture is never compromised.

Planks are another terrific lumbar stabilization exercise. In a plank, the patient lies prone and then props himself up on his elbows and toes so that his head, upper

G. Cooper, *Non-Operative Treatment of the Lumbar Spine*,
DOI 10.1007/978-3-319-21443-6_16

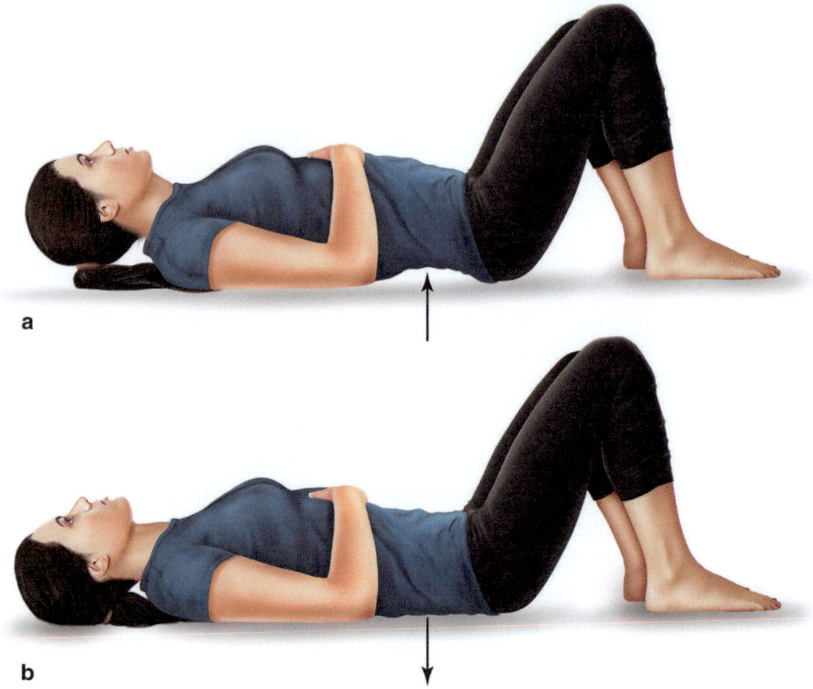

Fig. 16.1 Posterior pelvic tilt

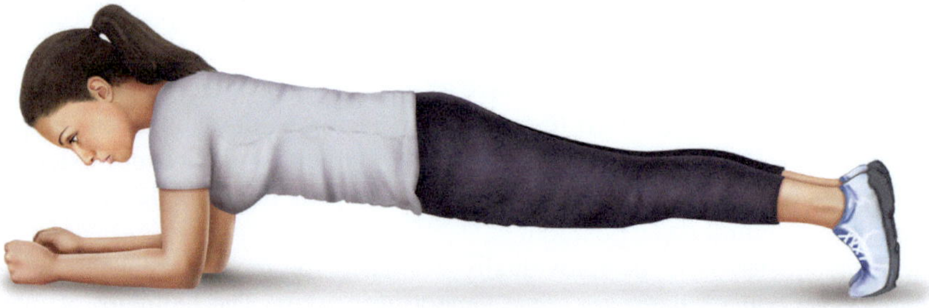

Fig. 16.2 Plank

back, lower back, and buttocks are in a straight line such that were a ruler to be placed on his back, it would remain completely straight (Fig. 16.2).

Once this exercise is easy for a patient to perform, variations are introduced such as side planks, and then the patient may progress to even more challenging variations such as dynamic planks. A dynamic plank involves holding a plank position and then taking away one or two of the supporting limbs but reaching for a predetermined spot. For example, a person may hold a plank position and then extend a hand 5 or 10 in. in front of him as if reaching for an object. Another variation may include raising a hand and contralateral leg and holding that position.

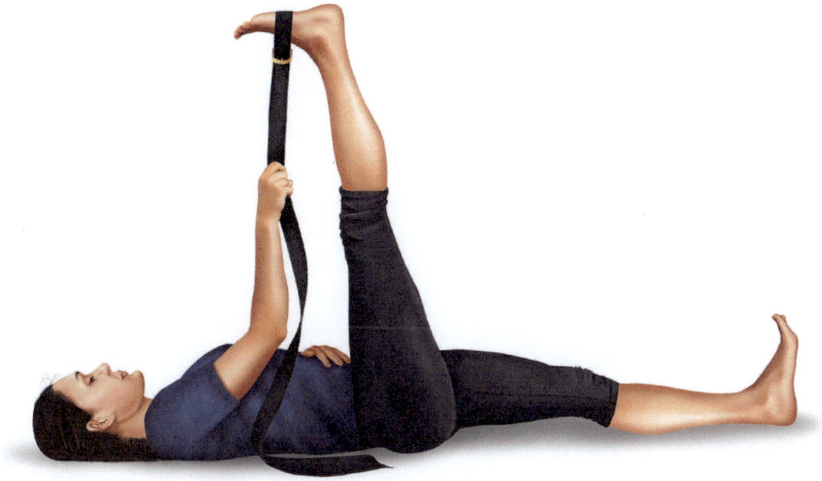

Fig. 16.3 Knee extensor stretch

Stretching the hip flexors is an important part of most therapeutic exercise programs for lower back problems. Recall that the hip flexor tendons attach to the transverse processes of the spine. When the hip flexors are tight (and they are often tight in people), they create a pulling torque on the spine, bringing it unhealthily forward. The hip flexors are a powerful muscle group and so this anterior torque can have very deleterious effects on the spine's health.

Knee extensor stretching is also often included in a back exercise program. The old-fashioned way of bending at the hips and trying to touch one's hands to the ground is not a good way to stretch the hamstrings as this places unnecessary and unwanted stress on the lower back. A preferred method to stretch the knee extensors is to have the patient lie on his back and then slowly bring his leg into the air. The patient may use a belt or rope to help bring his foot up. Ideally, while performing this stretch, the person can simultaneously perform a pelvic tilt, which serves the dual purpose of protecting the spine during the exercise and also strengthening the lumbar stabilizing muscles at the same time (Fig. 16.3).

In patients with flexion-biased pain, trunk extension stretches are very important. There are two common ways to perform trunk extension stretches. In one form, the patient is standing and places her hands on her hips as she arches her trunk backward until she feels a gentle stretch in the lower back. When she feels the stretch, she pauses and holds the position for 10–20 s. In another method to perform a trunk extension stretch, the patient lies in the prone position and slowly extends her back by coming up to her elbows until she feels the stretch and then she holds that position.

Chapter 17
The Mind-Body Connection: Is Stress Important?

As the decades have gone by, the role of stress and mental stability in a patient's life and the role that stress may play in a patient with lower back pain have become increasingly evident as a factor to always remember to consider. Dr. John Sarno did not invent the idea of somatization of stress as pain, but he certainly did a lot to popularize it and bring it to the awareness of patients and physicians alike. With his wildly popular book, *The Mind-Body Connection*, he introduced to the general population the concept (that he terms "tension myositis syndrome" or "TMS") that emotional stress can and often does become realized as physical pain.

The notion that stress "causes most back pain" is outdated and ignores decades of meticulous research that has revealed the most common spinal pain generators such as the facet joint, disc, and sacroiliac joint. However, most people—doctors and patients alike—would cede the principle that stress, just as sleep deprivation does, has the potential to make pain feel worse. A patient with discogenic lower back pain is likely to suffer more with that lower back pain if he also just lost his job and is going through a divorce. That is, seen through the prism of a large amount of stress in one's life, pain feels worse. Similarly, insomnia may magnify a patient's pain. Some patients have indeed been found to have *all* of their pain originate from the stress in their life, though this remains a very small minority of patients.

Most doctors who treat pain and take time to talk to their patients have stories about patients who broke down crying when they talked about something traumatic in their life. Once a patient opens up about a traumatic event, sometimes they immediately realize that their pain was alleviated by simply expressing and identifying their stress. The research on stress and its role in causing or exacerbating lower back symptoms is small and inconclusive. In this author's experience, patients who appear introspective and patients who wonder aloud if their stress is contributing to their pain typically may have stress as a component of their pain, but that component is likely to be a small component at most. Rather, it is the patient who abjectly denies that their recent divorce, loss of a job, loss of a parent, or other major emotional stress could possibly have anything to do with their pain—*it is precisely this patient* that is more likely to have a strong psychological component to his pain.

G. Cooper, *Non-Operative Treatment of the Lumbar Spine*,
DOI 10.1007/978-3-319-21443-6_17

Consider the following scenario. A doctor asks her patient, "Mr. Romero, you certainly do seem to have a lot of stress in your life. Do you think that your recent divorce and loss of your job may in some way be contributing to your pain?" If Mr. Romero were to respond, "No! What? Do you think I'm making this up? I'm in pain! Won't you help me? I'm not crazy!," it is this sort of response that should prompt concern that stress may be a significant portion of Mr. Romero's pain. This sort of closed response reflects a disconnect in Mr. Romero between his emotions and his awareness of how those emotions are likely interplaying with his body.

By contrast, if Mr. Romero were to respond, "Well, doctor, I've been thinking about that. I don't know. I certainly am stressed and I've tried to think if that is causing my pain but I really don't think so," he is clearly open to the idea that stress is playing a role in his pain. It is this response that reflects that Mr. Romero is more in touch with his feelings and how they may be affecting his overall health. Ironically, it is with this type of response that a strong psychological component to the pain is significantly less probable. Of course, to emphasize, the above is this author's professional opinion and is not grounded in evidence-based medicine.

In the end, it is important to treat the entire patient and not just the patient's spine. If stress is suspected, it is always appropriate and healthy to raise it as a question. If the patient is resistant to the suggestion, it is generally worth noting. A referral to a clinical psychologist or other mental health provider, if done in a tactful and non-threatening manner, may be very helpful to that patient.

Chapter 18
Alternative Treatments

There are a wide range of alternative treatments for spinal pathologies. Alternative should be defined here as treatments that lack a generally accepted standard of care by medical doctors based on a lack of rigorous scientific studies supporting their usage. When considering alternative treatments, it is important to always remember that lack of data to prove effectiveness is not the same thing as data proving ineffectiveness. That is to say that in many respects, the jury is still out in terms of evidence-based medicine when it comes to treatments such as acupuncture, chiropractic care, Feldenkrais, and other treatments.

Despite a lack of validation from evidence-based medicine, the usage of alternative treatments by patients with spinal pathologies is enormous. A busy spine specialist may have never seen a patient who has previously gone to a chiropractor or acupuncturist, but those patients have seen the spine specialist. That is to say that sometimes doctors remain unaware of their patients' usage of alternative medicine because the physician does not ask the question. In turn, many patients are reluctant to bring up their trials of alternative medicine because they may fear their physician will not approve. The disconnectedness between alternative medical practitioners and medical spine specialists has lessened over the decades but it persists, and it need not. Alternative medicine can play a productive role in treating patients, particularly if its usage is integrated into the overall treatment paradigm. When advising about alternative medicine, it is important that a patient understand what treatment is evidence-based medicine and what treatment is not. If that patient is going to pursue a treatment that is not evidence based, then ideally that treatment should first and foremost be unlikely to cause harm to that patient. Ideally, that treatment should not be painful or overly costly.

G. Cooper, *Non-Operative Treatment of the Lumbar Spine*,
DOI 10.1007/978-3-319-21443-6_18

Chiropractic Care

Perhaps the most common alternative treatment for lumbar spine pathologies is chiropractic care. The tradition of chiropractic medicine follows the tradition of practitioners known as bonesetter who can trace their lineage to ancient Egypt and Greece. Bonesetters were present in the 1800s in North America as well and gave rise in many respects to the field of osteopathy. In the 1890s Daniel David Palmer took those same principles of bonesetters and developed the field known as chiropractic medicine. Chiropractic care originally purported that the problems of the body originated from misalignment of the spine. A chiropractor in this school of thought may not be interested in a patient's "symptoms" because those symptoms originate from subluxations and misalignments of the spine. Therefore, a practitioner must only examine the spine and address that and the symptoms will essentially resolve on their own. Over the years, this traditional chiropractic school of thought has fallen out of favor, and today the vast majorities of chiropractors integrate use adjustments and manipulations to address musculoskeletal complaints and overall wellness, including in many instances ergonomic, nutritional, and lifestyle issues, but also seek to integrate their care with more traditional allopathic medical care. From an allopathic medical perspective, ideally chiropractic care can be used as a means to help address myofascial pain and adhesions and ultimately be one more tool to help enable a patient to return to therapeutic exercises. If exercises are not incorporated into a treatment program, chiropractic or otherwise, for lower back pain or radicular pain, then the likelihood is that the patient will need to continue to seek the chiropractic adjustments indefinitely as the patient actively strengthening and stretching the muscles surrounding the problem should be viewed as an integral part of most treatment paradigms.

Acupuncture

Apart from praying, acupuncture is one of, if not *the*, oldest known medical treatments. Some texts trace the use of some form of acupuncture back to the Bronze Age. What is certain is that the practice of acupuncture has existed in various forms for thousands of years. Indeed, the longevity of the treatment is often cited as implicit proof of its effectiveness. Of course, longevity of a treatment may make it intriguing, but it is not proof of usage. Over the years, evidence for acupuncture for a variety of pathologies such as postoperative nausea has been found. However, evidence for acupuncture in the use of various spinal pathologies is controversial at best. If acupuncture is to be considered evidence-based medicine for various spinal pathologies, then more research is certainly needed.

The basic philosophy behind acupuncture is that there are energy channels called meridians that flow through the body. It is the disruption of this energy that leads to symptoms and medical pathologies. Acupuncture uses points (called acupuncture points) in the body to access this energy (called chi) in order to re-equilibrate it. By balancing the energy, the symptoms in the body will take care of themselves. For this reason, a patient with lower back pain may be treated by an acupuncturist with only needles in that patient's ear or foot.

There are different schools of acupuncture and the specific approach will differ depending on the philosophy of the school. Schools differ based on geographic location such as Chinese versus Japanese versus Korean versus French, and then also within a given country, there will be different schools of acupuncture and differing approaches to practicing the art.

Anecdotally, there is no doubt that many patients report relief from acupuncture for a variety of problems, including spinal pathologies. When performed by an experienced, expert practitioner, acupuncture should be safe and is generally found to be at minimum a pleasant experience by most patients who pursue it. Some acupuncturists blend traditional acupuncture with a more allopathic approach. They can accomplish by placing acupuncture needles in muscles in spasm, effectively performing a dry needle trigger point maneuver of the muscle, and this may provide additional relief for some patients.

Prolotherapy

Prolotherapy is a treatment designed to promote the growth of normal cells and tissue. The theory behind prolotherapy of creating irritation in an effort to stimulate the body to heal itself is traced back to Roman times when gladiators were treated by using hot needles to stimulate healing around injured joints. Prolotherapy as we recognize its practice more today is traced back to the 1930s when an osteopathic surgeon named Dr. Earl Gedney treated his own injured and hypermobile thumb with an injectable sclerosing solution. His thumb was reportedly healed by this procedure and Dr. Gedney began experimenting with different sclerosing solutions and applications.

Essentially, prolotherapy involves the injection of a dextrose solution into the pathologic site. The idea is that the dextrose is irritating to the tissue, and this irritation and inflammation caused by the injection will stimulate increased vascular flow and a cascade of cellular events that results in the body healing itself. Over the years, the popularity of prolotherapy has waxed and waned. Despite its intermittent popularity as a treatment by medical and osteopathic doctors alike and despite certain self-reported success rates of 80–90 % by the physicians performing the procedure on their patients, the objective evidence for its usage in patients with lower back pain remains purely anecdotal and unconvincing. Still, when performed by an experienced physician, prolotherapy should be safe and some patients do report good outcomes.

Platelet-Rich Plasma

Driven in large part by its usage in recent years by high-profile athletes including Tiger Woods, Rafael Nadal, and Takashi Saito, platelet-rich plasma (PRP) has received a large amount of attention in the popular press as a potential treatment for all sorts of musculoskeletal maladies, including lower back pathologies. The principle of PRP is similar to prolotherapy. In PRP, blood is taken from a patient and then that blood is centrifuged in order to obtain a platelet-rich plasma. This platelet-rich plasma (PRP) is then injected into the site of pathology. The PRP has been shown to increase the concentration of growth factors. The theory is that this increased concentration of growth factors will then spur the patients' natural healing processes to heal the effected body part being treated. The anecdotal evidence for PRP (as was initially the case for prolotherapy) is tantalizing. Rigorous evidence-based trials for PRP have so far not shown efficacy for PRP for spinal pathologies, but many trials are ongoing. The idea of PRP is exciting, and an evidence-based role for PRP may indeed be found with further study. As of yet, the treatment remains experimental but based on anecdotal evidence as well as some histological studies that provide good concept rationale for why it *might* help some people. Excitement should remain somewhat tempered. One of the exciting roles for PRP was thought to be in strengthening tendons. However, a 2010 study of PRP for Achilles tendonitis showed no significant improvement over placebo [1]. Then again, a more recent study in 2012 found very significant improvement in chronic Achilles tendinosis being treated with PRP [2]. Studies on the use of PRP with rotator cuff tendon repair have likewise yielded mixed results [3, 4]. Many of the studies are limited with relatively small numbers of patients in specific pathologies. In one double-blind placebo-controlled study presented in 2013, patients with discogenic lower back pain were treated with intradiscal PRP or placebo and patients reported greater improvement and were more satisfied with the PRP treatment as compared with placebo [5]. Still, the sample size for this and other studies remain small and more research is needed. Ultimately, there may be a role for PRP in spinal pathologies, but further research will be needed to illuminate what any of those usages may include.

References and Suggested Further Reading

1. De Vos RJ, Weir A, van Schie HT, Bierma-Zeinstra SM, Verhaar JA, Weinans H, Tol JL. Platelet-rich plasma injection for chronic Achilles tendinopathy: a randomized controlled trial. JAMA. 2010;303(2):144–9.
2. Monto RR. Platelet rich plasma treatment for chronic Achilles tendinosis. Foot Ankle Int. 2012;33(5):379–85.
3. Barber FA, Hrnack SA, Snyder SJ, Hapa O. Rotator cuff repair healing influenced by platelet-rich plasma construct augmentation. Arthroscopy. 2011;27(8):1029–35.
4. Abtahi AM, Granger EK, Tashjian RZ. Factors affecting healing after arthroscopic rotator cuff tear. World J Orthop. 2015;6(2):211–20.
5. Terry A, Lutz G, et al. Lumbar intradiscal platelet rich plasma injections: a prospective, double-blind, randomized controlled trial (2013), International Spine Intervention Society – 2013 21st annual scientific meeting research abstracts. Pain Med. 2013;14:1269–76. doi:10.1111/pme.12219.

Part II
Clinical Scenarios

Any doctor who sees patients on a daily basis knows that many patients—most patients—don't fit neatly into a chapter. That is to say that patients' symptoms present in anomalous ways, have multifactorial pain patterns and other medical problems that can obscure the reason they are presenting in the first place, and generally present with a multitude of symptoms that are by their nature individualistic and sometimes difficult to characterize. Perhaps one of the greatest complaints levied at the doctrine of strict evidence-based medicine is that every patient is different, every patient has their own particular signs and symptoms as well as their own individual needs and expectations, and every patient must therefore be uniquely approached. As a result, applying a cookie-cutter style of medical practice to a complex and highly individualistic patient population can be challenging and at times even counterproductive.

It is into this constant and fluid tension between an evidence-based bedrock of knowledge and the highly individualized way in which each patient presents that the informed doctor walks and must make her way. This is the ever evolving challenge and beauty of medicine. In the end we physicians are scientists practicing an art form.

What follows in this section is a series of case scenarios pulled from actual case files of spine physicians. Each case is presented as the spine physician saw the patient and as such is at a different stage in diagnosis and treatment. After the patient is presented, the reader is asked to consider the next appropriate step. Following this consideration, a discussion of the pros and cons of the various next steps is discussed. The process then repeats itself until there is a resolution of the case. In this way, the reader may test himself to apply his knowledge to the clinical scenario.

Again, these are real patients (with identifying information obviously removed) and so the reader may consider himself the treating physician, sitting across from his patient, gathering the information, and planning a next step. The intent of this is to simulate, in a small way, a nonsurgical spine fellowship in which learned knowledge may be applied in real-world setting. Remember that the importance in evaluating a patient is not in knowing what the patient has or doesn't have as sometimes this is impossible to know without gathering more information.

Rather, the important thing is to have a process, an algorithm that can be applied so that the doctor knows how *to get to* an appropriate diagnosis and treatment. It is also important to know when a diagnosis or treatment path may deviate from evidence-based medicine because of an individual's particular circumstances. Armed with applied knowledge, a doctor's patients will always get comprehensive, detailed, measured care that is based in evidence and applied individually in the office. Let's get started.

Chapter 19
Clinical Case #1: James

James is an 84-year-old retired ironworker. He is referred by his primary care provider. James has a 10-year history of intermittent lower back pain that he says sometimes refers into the bilateral buttocks. The pain has been slowly getting worse in the last 2 years and finally he told his primary care doctor about it because the pain has been preventing him from going for walks, which is something he loves to do. He can walk about a block before the pain starts to get bad, and at a block and a half, James feels that he has to sit down because of the pain. The pain is much worse with standing and often he has no pain with sitting.

James' back feels very stiff in the morning, but he does some gentle stretching in the morning and that serves to get his back feeling looser and ready to start the day. He rates the pain while sitting as a 1/10 on VAS. He rates the pain as 8/10 on VAS after walking a block and says that the pain will get to a 10/10 if he continues to push it with walking. James says that one time he walked "too far" and ended up having to sit on the side of the road until the pain passed so that he could walk back home.

James takes Tylenol for his pain and says that it used to help but it does not anymore. He sometimes takes Aleve and finds it helps a little more than the Tylenol used to but he doesn't like taking medications. He has not done any physical therapy for the pain and has not had any other treatments, including no acupuncture or chiropractic care. He has had no imaging studies of his lower back.

In general, other than his back pain, James is in good medical health. He has high cholesterol and hypertension but these are managed well with medications. He has no history of cancer. James does some stretching in the morning for exercise. He has been doing the same stretches for about 20 years. He learned the stretches from his cousin who is a personal trainer. Besides his morning stretches, James does not exercise regularly but he does enjoy walking. It is his inability to walk due to the pain that has driven James to seek help for his lower back pain. James denies any radiating leg pain and denies any numbness, tingling, burning, or weakness in the legs.

G. Cooper, *Non-Operative Treatment of the Lumbar Spine*,
DOI 10.1007/978-3-319-21443-6_19

Physical Examination

On physical examination, James is 5′10 in., 185 lb. His gait is non-antalgic. He walks slightly stooped forward and has some mild thoracic kyphosis. He has full, pain-free lumbar trunk flexion but is restricted in lumbar extension and has pain with bilateral oblique lumbar extension.

James has good muscle tone and 5/5 strength in the lower extremities. He has a negative straight leg raise bilaterally, 2+ reflexes in the patella and Achilles, and no sensation deficits. His lumbar paraspinals are not tender and neither are his sacroiliac joints. He has a negative FABER test, which is a provocative maneuver designed to illicit sacroiliac joint pain. His hip flexors and knee extensors are very tight with passive range of motion. His hips have slightly restricted range of motion but no pain is produced with passive movement.

Assessment and Plan

Having heard James' presentation, what does he likely have and what is the next step that you would take as his treating physician?

James' age, history, and physical examination certainly leave the impression that he is likely suffering from facet joint pain. His pain is axial, worse with walking (trunk extension) and better with sitting (trunk flexion). He has no obvious radicular component, is neurologically intact, and has pain reproduced with extension of the trunk, particularly oblique extension which loads the facet joints.

While clinically these are all important points, it is important to remember that if we stick to the literature, it is still only about a 30 % probability that the pain is coming from the facet joints. There remains approximately a 40 % probability that the pain is coming from the intervertebral disc and 10–15 % chance that the pain is coming from the sacroiliac joints.

In the end, for James, our academic brain tells us that the pain is *most likely* discogenic in nature, then facet, and then sacroiliac joint and that the only way to figure out which is causing James' pain is to inject the structure and take away the pain. If the pain goes away, we found the source. If the pain does not go away, then we need to go onto the next structure. Our clinical brain should be telling us that everything James presents with *sounds* most like facet joint pain.

With those thoughts in tow, what do we do for James? Remember that James has not had any imaging studies and he has not tried any physical therapy. There are various appropriate ways of approaching James in this instance.

It would not be unreasonable to send James to physical therapy and see how he does after 4–6 weeks. Depending on James' preference, it would also not be unreasonable to order an MRI and, assuming no surprises on the MRI, consider performing a medial branch block or facet joint injection to aid in the diagnosis and possibly jump-start the treatment process.

All of the above was discussed with James. James wanted to approach things as conservatively as possible. He did not like taking medications and wanted injections to be performed "only if absolutely necessary." As such, an MRI of the lumbar spine was ordered and James was sent to physical therapy.

The prescription for physical therapy included the use of soft tissue mobilization, other manual techniques, ultrasound, heat, ice, and electrical stimulation as needed and a focus on lumbar stabilizing exercises with a flexion bias and hip flexor stretching and knee extensor stretching.

Follow-Up

James had his MRI and went to physical therapy for 4 weeks. He followed up 5 weeks after his initial visit. James' MRI of the lumbar spine revealed a grade I L4–L5 anterolisthesis, multilevel facet joint arthropathy, and degenerative disc disease as well as an L2–L3 disc herniation. Clinically, James reported good progress after 4 weeks of therapy. Overall he felt he was 30 % improved in terms of pain. James was able to walk almost a block and a half before the pain became bad enough to make him want to sit down. He felt stronger and his posture was improved. His MRI findings were reviewed with him. Given his improvement, what is the most appropriate next step?

A good general rule of thumb is that if a patient is Y percentage better on day 30 than he was on day 1, then he has every reason to believe that he will continue to improve at that rate such that on day 60 he may be 2Y better than on day 1. So, for James, since he is 30 % better after 1 month of physical therapy, it is reasonable to think he may be 60 % better after another month of physical therapy.

If James were frustrated with his progress and wanted to speed up his improvement, it would not be unreasonable to consider a medial branch block or other intervention at that time. However, James was happy with his improvement and wanted to continue with physical therapy. As such, James returned to physical therapy for another month. He returned for another follow-up 4 weeks later and reported 70 % overall improvement. After 2 months of physical therapy, James reported being able to walk about two and a half blocks before the pain started to get bad enough to where he felt he had to sit down. James wanted to try 1 more month of physical therapy. As he was making steady improvement, it was agreed that this seemed like the best course of action.

James followed up after another month of physical therapy. Unfortunately, James did not improve since the previous visit. He still felt about 70 % improved overall. He could walk about two and a half blocks before the pain got bad, and he also felt that if he paused at two blocks and did some stretches, then he could continue walking for an even longer period of time. Overall, James was very happy with his progress and his ability to stand and go for a walk. James had learned his therapeutic exercises from physical therapy and he was able to perform the exercises at his home.

At this time, it was explained to James that he had multiple treatment options. James could continue his home exercise program which would hopefully maintain his progress and possibly slowly improve his symptoms. Alternatively, if the pain were still limiting to him, additional interventions could be considered starting most likely with medial branch blocks or intra-articular injections of the facet joints. James did not feel the need to pursue further intervention. He was frankly happy with the way his back was feeling. He felt stronger than he had in a long time and did not feel that his quality of life would be significantly improved for what he wanted to do—even if he were able to get the last 30 % of his pain to go away. As such, James was discharged to continue his home exercises and would call if the symptoms were to worsen.

James returned a year later with a completely different problem in his neck. As far as his lumbar spine was concerned, he reported that in the intervening year, his lower back and buttock pain continued to be well controlled with his home exercise program which he performed about 15 min at a time, five times per week.

James' case serves a few valuable points. Because James did as well as he did with physical therapy, the actual source of James' pain will have to remain a point of conjecture as his symptoms never merited performing the gold standard diagnostic test of an injection to find the source of pain. However, in James' case, the lack of a definitive diagnosis should not be seen as a defeat. Quite to the contrary, James' pain resolved to the point that he did not feel limited by the pain. In short, James was happy with his results from a very conservative intervention of physical therapy. If James had been dissatisfied with his pain level and tolerance for exercise following physical therapy, it would likely have been appropriate and important to perform additional steps to diagnose and treat his pain. However, if James has no interest in walking for longer without pain and if James is perfectly content to walk two and a half blocks before resting, then there is no need to go any further because James' goals have been met.

Chapter 20
Clinical Case #2: Ruth

Ruth is a 64-year-old married attorney who presents with a 7-month history of right-sided lower back and buttock pain. She is being referred to this office by her physical therapist. She had been sent to her physical therapist by her primary care doctor. After 15 sessions of physical therapy, her therapist told her that because she was not making any progress with therapy, she should see a specialist.

Ruth's pain started without any inciting event that she can recall. She notes that the pain started insidiously and then progressively got worse to the point that in the last 4 months, Ruth has trouble performing her activities of daily living because of the intensity of the pain. Ruth's pain is worst with standing and better with sitting. The pain is worse in the morning and also worse with transitioning from sit to stand if she has been sitting for a prolonged period of time.

Ruth's pain does not radiate into the legs and she denies any numbness, tingling, or subjective weakness in the legs. Ruth says that she can walk about two city blocks before the pain reaches 8/10 on VAS and makes her want to sit down. She has not had any radiologic studies of her lumbar spine.

Ruth has been taking 800 mg of ibuprofen three times per day and says that this helps her pain but it upsets her stomach and she would like to stop taking it. She has tried Tylenol for the pain in the past but this has never helped her. Ruth did go to a chiropractor three times but this did not help her symptoms at all so she stopped going. Ruth notes that moist heat makes the pain feel better temporarily but then the pain keeps returning.

Ruth has a past medical history of high blood pressure that is managed with hydrochlorothiazide and otherwise does not take any medications other than the ibuprofen. Ruth notes that she does not exercise regularly and says that her hours are so long at work that it has been years since she had a regular work-out routine.

G. Cooper, *Non-Operative Treatment of the Lumbar Spine*,
DOI 10.1007/978-3-319-21443-6_20

Physical Examination

On physical examination, Ruth is 5′4″ and 130 lb. Her gait is normal. She has full, pain-free trunk flexion but is restricted in trunk extension and has pain and restricted movement with right oblique extension of her lumbar spine. She has a negative straight leg raise bilaterally. Ruth's right lumbar paraspinals are diffusely tender but no specific trigger points can be identified. Her right sacroiliac joint is tender. She has a negative FABER test.

Ruth has 5/5 strength in her lower extremities bilaterally. Her sensation is intact and her patella and Achilles reflexes are 1+ bilaterally.

Assessment and Plan

Having heard Ruth's presentation, what does she likely have and what is the next step that you would take as her treating physician?

Ruth has chronic right lower back pain. It is helpful to review some of the pertinent points. Ruth is over 60. Her pain is axial and non-radiating. She has no neurologic signs or symptoms. Her pain is worse with standing (trunk extension) and is better with sitting (trunk flexion). On physical examination, Ruth's pain is easily reproduced with right oblique extension of her lumbar spine. All of these important points suggest that Ruth's pain is emanating from her facet joints.

Indeed, based on her history and physical examination, she certainly seems to have relatively classic facet joint pain. However, recall that this is a clinical assessment, and in fact it is important—some might say critical—to remember that the most likely diagnosis for Ruth's pain based on epidemiology is discogenic pain (about 40 % of the time) followed by facet joint pain (about 30 % of the time) and then sacroiliac joint pain (10–15 % of the time).

Ruth has not had any radiologic studies of her lumbar spine yet. Based on the fact that she has had the pain for 7 months and is likely going to require interventional procedures for diagnosis and possible treatment, after a full discussion and explanation of her options, it is agreed that Ruth should first have an MRI of the lumbar spine without contrast.

Follow-Up

Ruth gets the MRI scan and returns for follow-up. Her MRI reveals multilevel facet joint arthropathy and a small central disc herniation at L5–S1. Ruth's MRI findings are reviewed with her and it is explained to her that her MRI is essentially "average" or "normal for her age." Another way of explaining this is to say that if one took an MRI of one hundred people who were Ruth's age and had never had a pain in their lumbar spine and if one then compared these asymptomatic normal subjects' MRIs with Ruth's MRI, it would be impossible to know who has symptoms and who does not. It is important to explain to Ruth that this is not to diminish her pain or suggest that it is "made up." Ruth's MRI is consistent with her pain and important to consider, but in and of itself is not diagnostic of what is causing her particular pain. The MRI is, to be more succinct, one piece of the puzzle.

Given that Ruth's pain is significantly interfering with her quality of life and that she has not improved with physical therapy, it is elected to perform a diagnostic facet joint block of her right L3–4, L4–5, and L5–S1 facet joints. Ruth understands that epidemiologically her most likely pain source is the disc; however, she is clinically most consistent with facet joint pain (1), and a diagnostic block of the facet joints is much less invasive than an epidural steroid injection (2). For these reasons, the facet joint block is performed for diagnostic as well as hopefully therapeutic purposes.

It was agreed to perform an intra-articular facet joint injection procedure in the hopes of providing lasting pain relief as well as serving to help confirm the diagnosis. Importantly, intra-articular facet joint injections in and of themselves have not been shown to provide lasting pain relief. However, if the facet joints are found to be the source of the pain and if the inflammation is adequately reduced for a significant period of time with the steroid in the injection, then ideally the patient can use the injection as a window of opportunity in order for her to do her physical therapy exercises, which in turn help improve her biomechanics and unload the spine so that the same daily biomechanical stresses are no longer passing through the same facet joints. By reducing the biomechanical load on the facet joints, the hope and plan is that the inflammation and pain do not return.

After the facet joint injection, Ruth is given a pain diary to record her pain relief for the following 8 h after the injection. A quick note on pain diaries is that it is important to give clear, precise instructions when handing out a pain diary to a patient. If Ruth were to go home after the injection and take a nap (as has been known to happen), then the diagnostic aspect of the facet joint injection would have been wasted because of course Ruth would not have any pain while sleeping. It is important that Ruth understands *why* the injection is being performed and what is being asked of her.

Ruth is instructed to stand and walk in order to see if the pain is really better. Ruth records her pain improvement (or lack thereof) at 1 min postinjection, 20 min postinjection, 1 h postinjection, and then every hour after that for a total of 8 h. Before Ruth leaves the office, she fills out the first time interval for the pain diary which is at 1 min. At 1 min, Ruth stands and says she thinks she feels "a very little bit better." She rates the improvement at 10 %.

Ruth returns for a follow-up visit 2 weeks after having the facet joint injection. She brings her pain diary and the results are discussed. Ruth reported a 10 % pain improvement for 1 h and then the pain returned to baseline. At 2 weeks, the steroids had also done nothing for her and she was still at her baseline pain.

The 10 % improvement that Ruth experienced is not meaningful for the purposes of the pain diary. If the pain relief is not at least 80 % improvement, then it is largely considered a negative result. The patient should not have to guess or think too hard about whether the pain is better. The improvement to the patient should be profound and obvious. Recall too that it is important to instruct the patient to report whether or not the pain is completely better in one part of the back and not at all better in a different part. If that happens, it may be that overall the patient feels about 10 % better, but if 100 % of the superior part of the pain is gone and 90 % of the inferior part of the pain remains, then that is important to write down as the conclusion would be that the facet joints were likely causing the superior part of the pain but not the inferior part. In any event, in Ruth's case the pain did not improve other than a very mild 10 % for about an hour.

As the facet joint block did not result in any significant pain relief, the facet joint is ruled out as a potential pain generator for Ruth's pain. As a next step, because it is a less invasive procedure and because there is a large minority chance (10–15 %) that it is the pain generator, a right sacroiliac joint injection is performed for diagnostic as well as potentially therapeutic purposes.

Following the right sacroiliac joint injection, Ruth is again given a pain diary. This time when Ruth fills the pain diary out at 1 min, she reports 90 % pain relief. Ruth returns in 2 weeks again and reviews her pain diary as well as her overall improvement at 2 weeks.

For the pain diary, Ruth reported 90 % pain relief at 1 min, 20 min, and 1 h. At 2 h, she reported 80 % pain relief. At 3 and 4 h, she reported 70 % pain relief and at 5 h she reported 50 % pain relief. At 6 h her pain had returned to baseline and it stayed that way through 8 h.

At first Ruth was disappointed that the pain had returned after 8 h but she remembered that it may take several days or up to 2 weeks for the steroids to begin to work. In fact, 2 days after the sacroiliac joint injection, Ruth again started to feel better. At her follow-up appointment 2 weeks after the sacroiliac joint injection, Ruth reported that she was feeling 85 % improved.

Ruth's response is typical of a positive response to a sacroiliac joint injection. The reason she felt better for 4 h and then the pain returned soon after that is because the lidocaine had numbed the sacroiliac joint but then wore off after that time. The reason that Ruth felt better 2 days later was because it usually takes around 2–7 days for the steroids in an injection like this to reduce the targeted inflammation. The effects of the steroids typically crescendo over about 2 weeks. Some people do not see any improvement from the steroids until 2 weeks after an injection. It is because of this delayed onset of action for the steroids that the follow-up appointment is typically scheduled 2 weeks after an injection if steroids have been injected. In this way, the full effect—or most of the full effect—of the steroid can be seen so that a next step can be planned.

At 2 weeks, Ruth was delighted with her response to the sacroiliac joint injection. Because of her response, the sacroiliac joint was presumed to be the pain generator. Ruth's doctor reminded her that there was still a chance that she had experienced a false-positive reaction to the injection, but it certainly was most likely at that point that her pain was coming from the sacroiliac joint. Now that she was feeling better, Ruth was sent back to physical therapy with the purpose of learning a set of exercises to get the last 15 % of her pain to go away and stay away.

Ruth's return to physical therapy proved much more successful than her first time with therapy. For one, she now had a diagnosis that enabled the physical therapist to focus her efforts with Ruth on treating her sacroiliac joint. For another, now that the pain was not limiting Ruth from participating with the exercises, she was able to do more within the physical therapy. Over the next month, Ruth was able to become pain-free with physical therapy.

Ruth returned for a follow-up visit 18 months after the sacroiliac joint injection. Ruth reported that the pain had returned 4 months prior and had been getting progressively worse over the last 4 months. Ruth reported that she had learned her home exercise program from her physical therapist and that she had done those exercises for about 2 months after she was last seen in this office, but then she admitted that she had stopped doing her exercises because she "was feeling fine" and life was very busy between her work obligations and family life.

Her pain over the last 4 months felt exactly how it had felt when she first presented with right lower back and buttock pain. Ruth had tried to return to doing her physical therapy exercises but the pain had only gotten worse and now was too intense for her to do the exercises anyway. Ruth was taking ibuprofen 800 mg PO TID and that was barely helping her pain and it was upsetting her stomach. Based on the fact that her symptoms were the same as they were previously and based on the fact that her symptoms were limiting her ability to participate with her therapeutic exercises, it was elected to inject Ruth's right sacroiliac joint again.

Ruth was given her pain diary again after the sacroiliac joint injection and again she had about 4 h of 90 % pain relief followed by a return of her pain. Again it took a little over 2 days for the pain to go away again. At her 2-week follow-up appointment, again she was 85 % pain-free.

Now that she was feeling so much better, Ruth was sent back to physical therapy to review and refine her home exercise program. One of the things that Ruth had said when she returned with her recurrent pain was that one of the reasons she had stopped the physical therapy home exercise program in the first place was that it was taking her too long to complete it. When asked how long she had been doing the exercises per night, Ruth said it took her about 40 min. This time, when she returned to physical therapy, Ruth knew that she had to leave physical therapy with a more abbreviated home exercise program that she would realistically be able to do consistently on her own long after the pain was in her rear-view mirror.

Ruth's failure to continue with her home exercise program after the initial injection and physical therapy brings up a useful teaching point. It is much more important for patients to perform a consistent home exercise program of 10–15 min a day than for them to have a 40 or 60 min home exercise program that they might do once per week but likely won't do at all once the pain has been absent for several months.

In general, it is a good idea for patients to be sure to have two home exercise programs—one that is approximately 10 min long and one that is approximately 40 min long. If the patient feels ambitious on a certain day then she can and should do the longer program. However, she should not do the longer program at the expense of doing the shorter program every day or *at least* five times per week. That is to say that the more home exercises the better, but consistency of performance is paramount for ultimate success.

Ideally, too, the patient's home exercise program becomes integrated into a more robust overall home exercise system that incorporates cardiovascular exercises and general stretching and strength training. However, again, in terms of addressing the particular issue (sacroiliac joint pain in Ruth's case), the most important thing is to be consistent with a 10 or 15 min home exercise program that is performed on a daily basis. If Ruth chooses to occasionally do a 40 min workout for her back or even an hour workout for her back, then that is icing on the cake.

Chapter 21
Clinical Case #3: Steve

Steve is a 22-year-old first-year graduate student in molecular biology who was referred by his friend. Steve has a 6-week history of right lower back pain, right buttock pain, and radiating right leg pain. The pain began without any particular inciting event that he can identify. The pain radiates from the right lower back and buttock into the right posterior thigh, lateral thigh, calf, and into the right dorsum of the foot. Steve's right lateral lower leg feels numb to him.

Steve's pain got much worse 1 week ago after a long car ride. In general, Steve says that his pain is worse with sitting and better with standing and/or walking. For the last week, since the long car ride, Steve has had trouble sleeping because he has trouble finding a comfortable position when lying down. A few times, the pain has woken him from sleep. When he sits for more than a few minutes, he rates the pain as 9/10 on VAS. He says the pain is also generally worse in the morning when he first wakes up.

Steve has been taking ibuprofen and acetaminophen but these medications have not been helping. He has trouble studying because of the pain. He does not feel as though his leg is weak. He has no changes in bowel or bladder habits. Upon closer questioning, Steve does recall an intermittent history of lower back pain and occasional right leg pain over the last 2 years since a long airplane ride, but he is quick to emphasize that the symptoms had always been very mild and so he did not take much notice of them.

Steve likes to work out and exercise although since starting graduate school he reports that he has not found time to go to the gym. Steve has no imaging studies of his lumbar spine and has not had any treatments for his back other than the over-the-counter medications that he has been taking.

G. Cooper, *Non-Operative Treatment of the Lumbar Spine*,
DOI 10.1007/978-3-319-21443-6_21

Physical Examination

On physical examination, Steve is 5′10″ and 180 lb. He has a normal gait. He has pain with trunk flexion at about 30°. He has full and pain-free lumbar extension but has moderate pain with right lumbar oblique extension. He has a positive straight leg raise at 40° and a positive right slump test.

Steve has 5/5 strength in the lower extremities except he has 5−/5 strength in his right EHL and right hip abductors. His sensation is intact to light touch. He has 2+ reflexes in the bilateral patella reflexes and 2+ in the left Achilles but 1+ in the right Achilles. His lumbar paraspinals are tender diffusely on the right side from L3 through S1. He has no tenderness over the right sacroiliac joint and he has a negative FABER test.

Assessment and Plan

Having heard Steve's presentation, what does he likely have and what is the next step that you would take as his treating physician?

Steve's presentation is very consistent with and perhaps classic for a right L5 and S1 radiculopathy. The fact that he has pain in an L5 and S1 distribution and positive dural tension signs points strongly toward the diagnosis. The fact that Steve has objective weakness in the right L5 myotome and decreased Achilles reflex (an S1 reflex) confirms the diagnosis and is concerning in its own right, meriting prompt attention and intervention.

After discussing his signs, symptoms, and likely pathophysiology, Steve is given a Medrol dose pack, gabapentin 100 mg PO TID, and an MRI of the lumbar spine without contrast is ordered.

Follow-Up

Steve returns 1 week later after having gotten his MRI. He reports that his pain was "much better" for 2 days with the Medrol dose pack but now his symptoms are back to baseline. He does not feel that the gabapentin is helping him, nor does he feel tired while taking the gabapentin.

Steve's MRI is reviewed with him. He has a large right L5–S1 paracentral disc herniation creating lateral recess stenosis and right L5–S1 foraminal stenosis. Given the subjective numbness and weakness, objective weakness, large disc herniation in the anatomical region that is consistent with his symptoms, his lack of response to gabapentin and a Medrol dose pack, and the fact that Steve does not feel he could tolerate physical therapy at his current level of symptoms, it is decided to perform a right L5 and S1 transforaminal epidural steroid injection.

Steve responds very well to the transforaminal epidural steroid injection. He returns for follow-up 2 weeks after the injection and reports 70 % reduction in pain and a resolution of his numbness. His physical examination is largely unchanged except that his straight leg raise is now positive at 60° and his overall pain with maneuvers is much reduced. His weakness is unchanged. Steve is sent to physical therapy to focus on extension-biased lumbar stabilization exercises as well as hip abductor strengthening.

Steve returns 6 weeks later and reports resolution of his symptoms. His physical examination is normal with no strength deficits, normal reflexes bilaterally, and negative dural tension signs (negative straight leg raise and negative slump test). Steve has learned his home exercise program and has begun to perform his exercises at home. He says it takes him 20 min to do his exercises and he enjoys doing them.

Steve is feeling good but he is concerned about his disc herniation and wonders what it means for his future prognosis. He asks if he should have a repeat MRI to see if the disc herniation has resolved. It is explained to Steve that a follow-up MRI of his lumbar spine is not indicated, necessary, or particularly important for that matter. Whether or not the disc herniation has resorbed, the treatment recommendations for Steve would be the same.

Once someone like Steve has had an episode of radiculopathy, it is more likely that he will have a similar episode in the future as compared with his age cohort. This would be true whether or not his disc herniation had reabsorbed. However, if Steve takes this experience as a learning opportunity to learn a set of home exercises (as he already has), if he continues to perform those exercises (as he intends), and if he learns to optimize his ergonomics at home and at work, then he is likely to have less of a chance of developing a recurrence of pain or other lumbar problems in the future as compared with his age cohort. It truly does become a glass half empty or half full scenario depending on the perspective. The point being that most people are at risk to some extent of developing a lower back problem. Most people could *probably* avoid a back problem if they performed a set of home exercises for their lumbar spine. However, most people don't do that until they have a problem. With Steve's motivation to perform his exercises, he may in fact be less likely to have a problem in the future than his age cohort.

Chapter 22
Clinical Case #4: Carol

Carol is a 52-year-old hairdresser. She has been referred by her primary care doctor because she has been having pain and weakness in her left leg. Carol works long hours and the more she stands, the worse the pain becomes. She says that she has had intermittent left lower back pain "for several years," but in the last year she has noted increased pain radiating into the left lower extremity. She says that she hates complaining about herself but that she does find that she has trouble getting through the day because of the pain. By the end of the day, her left leg and foot often feel numb and tingling.

Carol reports that she has noticed that she has been having problems with her balance, and at least 3 times in the last month, she has tripped over her left foot and almost fallen. She rates the pain as 2/10 at best while sitting and resting and 9/10 on VAS by the end of the day or if she has to stand for more than 30 min without taking a break.

Carol has been taking four Advil three times per day for at least 2 months, but she does not find it particularly helpful. The Advil does not bother her stomach. She has not tried taking Tylenol. She went to her primary care doctor for her regular checkup, and her primary care doctor told her she needs to be seen immediately for her lower back and leg problems. She has not had any imaging studies. Carol does not believe that her weakness in her leg is getting worse, but she is not sure and she does note that her three trips over her left foot were all within the last month and she does not remember tripping prior to that. The pain, though, has not been getting worse in the last few months.

Carol has not gone to physical therapy or had any other treatments for the left leg symptoms. She says that she works 6 days per week and looks forward to her 1 day off so she can lie in her bed with her feet up. In this position she is the most comfortable and can get some rest. She says that she does not have the time or energy to go to the gym. She used to like to walk in the mornings before work but she has not been able to do that for "at least a year" because of the pain.

G. Cooper, *Non-Operative Treatment of the Lumbar Spine*,
DOI 10.1007/978-3-319-21443-6_22

Physical Examination

On physical examination, Carol is 5′9″ and 140 lb. She has an antalgic Trendelenburg gait. She has full, pain-free lumbar trunk flexion, but she is restricted in lumbar extension and immediately gets severe left leg pain with minimal amount of left lumbar oblique extension. She has a positive straight leg raise on the left at 40°, and she has a positive straight leg raise on the right that reproduces her left leg symptoms. She has a positive slump test on the left.

Carol's sensation reveals decreased sensation to light touch in the left lateral lower leg and left dorsum of the foot. She has 4/5 left hip abductor strength, 4+/5 left dorsiflexor strength, 4+/5 left extensor hallucis longus, and 4+/5 left plantar flexor strength. She has no reflex in the left Achilles but otherwise has 2+ bilateral reflexes.

Carol has minimal tenderness in the left lumbar paraspinals and over the left sacroiliac joint. She has a negative FABER test. She has full and pain-free range of motion in her hips. She has relatively tight hip flexors and knee extensors.

Assessment and Plan

Having heard Carol's presentation, what does she likely have and what is the next step that you would take as her treating physician?

Carol's presentation is concerning for many features. She has significant pain and numbness as well as what appears to be progressive weakness based on the fact that she has been tripping in the last month. She has positive dural tension signs, including a straight leg raise on the right that reproduces her left leg symptoms, and she has decreased sensation and significant weakness in the L5 and S1 myotome distributions. She has no bowel or bladder changes so it is not an emergency, but diagnostics should be obtained with a great sense of urgency and treatment should be started as soon as possible.

Carol's symptoms and likely pathophysiology is discussed with her. Carol is reluctant to take a Medrol dose pack because she took one several years ago as a treatment for poison ivy and she says it made her "crazy." She agrees to go the next day for an MRI of the lumbar spine without contrast.

Follow-Up

Carol returns 2 days later with MRI in hand. Her MRI reveals a large lateral L5–S1 disc herniation impinging on the left L5 and S1 nerve roots. The MRI is reviewed with Carol and the different treatment options are presented to her. She agrees to undergo a left L5 and S1 transforaminal epidural steroid injection. The procedure is performed on the same day. She tolerates the procedure very well and is amazed to note that she has 100 % pain relief from the lidocaine in the injectate.

It is explained to Carol that her response to the lidocaine in the injection is good because it confirms the diagnosis but that she should expect that the pain is going to return once the lidocaine wears off in a few hours. Sure enough, 4 h after the injection, Carol's pain returns. Carol is also prescribed Lyrica 75 mg PO to be taken once at bedtime for 7 days and then BID if she tolerates it. She is also prescribed meloxicam 15 mg PO daily to be taken instead of the Advil that she has been taking.

Because of Carol's schedule and also because the pain is too intense to do much in terms of exercises, it is elected to hold off on physical therapy until the pain has reduced to the point that she would be able to tolerate more of the exercises.

Carol returns in 2 weeks and notes that the pain is 30 % improved. She tried taking the Lyrica but it made her very dizzy so she stopped taking it. She has been taking the meloxicam but does not feel it is helping her. On physical examination, the only change is that she no longer has a positive reverse straight leg raise. However, she continues to have a left straight leg raise positive at 50°, and her strength and sensation exam is unchanged as is the fact that she has no reflex in the left Achilles. It is elected to repeat the left L5 and S1 transforaminal epidural steroid injection.

Again, after the left L5 and S1 transforaminal epidural steroid injection, she has 100 % pain relief from the lidocaine in the injection. Carol is given a prescription for physical therapy and she agrees to start physical therapy in a week if the pain continues to improve. Carol returns in 2 weeks but this time the news is not good. The pain did not improve after the last injection and in fact she feels as if overall her pain has regressed to her baseline before the first injection. A repeat physical examination is performed and found to be unchanged from 2 weeks prior.

Carol is very upset and discouraged and she breaks down in the doctor's office and begins to cry saying that she is just "so tired of the pain." She just wants to be able to get through her day without crippling pain, and she is getting worried about the weakness in her leg which she says she is now more aware of than previous.

Given her lack of response to two epidural steroid injections, her MRI, and her neurologic loss, it is elected to refer Carol to a spine surgeon so that Carol gets a full understanding of her surgical options. Carol is not a surgical emergency. She does not have progressive neurologic loss. She does, however, have persistent neurologic loss and a recent history of progressive neurologic loss over the previous month. She also has severe pain that is significantly limiting her activities of daily living and her ability to exercise. She has not responded to two epidural steroid injections and so a third injection is unlikely to make a significant difference.

It is important to recognize that Carol still has conservative options including physical therapy, various pain medications, and chiropractic care, not to mention acupuncture and other modalities. However, given Carol's MRI, she would likely benefit from a relatively minor decompressive surgery and this may be her best option to get past the pain and back to her life sooner than later. Surgery does not guarantee a return of neurologic function, but intuitively it is understood that the sooner the neurologic loss is productively addressed, the better. Further, the sooner her pain is addressed the better.

Carol sees a local neurosurgeon who presents her surgical option of a discectomy and laminectomy. Carol is very comfortable with the neurosurgeon and does not feel the need to get a second surgical opinion. She calls her nonsurgical interventional spine doctor and the options are discussed on the phone. Carol goes ahead with the surgery.

Immediately following the surgery, Carol's pain is 95 % better. Over the course of the next 8 months, Carol learns a home exercise program of lumbar stabilizing exercises from her physical therapist, and sure enough her strength and sensation slowly return to normal. Carol was very nervous about the thought of surgery but is glad to have had it done and grateful that she was exposed sooner than later to that option.

Chapter 23
Clinical Case #5: Tania

Tania is a 52-year-old project manager with a 30-year history of chronic lower back and buttock pain. She recently changed primary care doctors and her new primary care doctor suggested that she come to this office. Tania reports that her pain began shortly after she had her first child at the age of 22. Since then, Tania has had another child and slowly over the last 30 years the pain in her lower back and buttock has gotten worse.

In the last 10 years, Tania's pain has been relatively constant. The pain is sharp and burning and drives Tania "crazy all the time." The pain is worse with any static position but is particularly worse with sitting and with transitioning from sit to stand after she has been sitting for more than a few minutes. Tania's pain does not radiate into the legs. She denies any numbness, tingling, or burning in the lower extremities and she does not believe that she has any weakness in the lower extremities.

Over the years, Tania has seen many doctors about her lower back pain. She has been to physical therapy for several months in the past but did not feel that was helpful except she liked the massages and the electrical stimulation "but the relief never lasted." She has been to chiropractors through the years and has found that manipulations sometimes help "for a couple of days" but the pain always returns.

Tania has had three epidural steroid injections that did not help at all. She is not sure what type of epidural steroid injections they were (interlaminar versus caudal versus transforaminal) and she is not sure at what level they were performed. Her last epidural steroid injection was 4 years ago. She has had "lots of trigger point injections" over the years and she usually finds that they help "for about a week" but the pain has always recurred.

Tania has had facet joint injections that did not help and she has had non-image-guided sacroiliac joint injections that did not help. Her last injection of any sort was 4 years ago. She does not remember ever being given a pain diary after any injection and is not sure what a pain diary means as no one has ever discussed it with her.

Over the last 4 years, Tania has been taking oxycodone 10 mg PO QID. She says that she hates needing pain medication and would love to get off of it but the oxycodone is the only thing that helps her get through the day. At night, she often takes

G. Cooper, *Non-Operative Treatment of the Lumbar Spine*,
DOI 10.1007/978-3-319-21443-6_23

cyclobenzaprine 10 mg in addition to the oxycodone to help her sleep. Without the medications, she says that she could not function. Tania has tried various nonsteroidal anti-inflammatory medications, both over the counter and by prescription, but she says that the only one that ever helped was Vioxx and that is unfortunately no longer available.

Tania's last imaging study was 5 years ago. She had an MRI at that time that revealed diffuse disc bulges and multilevel facet joint arthropathy. She has been to three different spine surgeons 4 years ago when she thought she could not take the pain anymore and just wanted "to fix the problem." Each surgeon that she saw recommended against any surgical intervention. After talking to the last spine surgeon, and after all of the failed previous treatments, she says that she basically accepted the status quo of pain and takes the pain medications to help get through her days and nights. She is very unhappy with the way her pain affects her and the way it limits her life and diminishes her quality of life, but from the conversations she has had with her doctors, she believes that there is nothing else that can help her. As she discusses it, Tania begins to cry. She says that her previous primary care doctor told her that she needs to accept the pain and take the pain medication as little as possible to get through the day.

Tania used to see a pain management specialist but she has been stable on her medications for 3 years and so for the last 2 years it is her primary care doctor who has written her pain medication prescriptions. Her new primary care doctor said that he was okay with writing the pain prescriptions if necessary but that hopefully something better could be found to treat her pain.

Tania rates the pain as 5/10 on VAS at best and 10/10 at worst. She says that she has 9/10 pain for at least a few hours every day. Other than her lower back and buttock pain, she has no significant medical history. She says that she knows she is overweight but has trouble losing the weight because her activity is so restricted because of the pain. Also, when she gets very stressed about the pain or upset about her life, she finds that she eats more than she would like. She says that she is generally a "happy person" but that the pain has been "overwhelming."

Physical Examination

On physical examination, Tania is 5′3″ and 150 lb. Tania has a normal gait although she is clearly in pain with transition from sit to stand. She has pain and restricted range of motion with trunk flexion, extension, and bilateral oblique extension. She has a negative straight leg raise bilaterally. Her lumbar paraspinals are diffusely tender. Her bilateral sacroiliac joints are tender. She has very tender quadratus lumborum muscles bilaterally but no actual trigger point with a referral pain pattern. She has a positive FABER test bilaterally.

Tania has 5/5 strength in her lower extremities bilaterally. She has intact sensation in her lower extremities bilaterally. She has 2+ reflexes in her patella and Achilles bilaterally.

Her MRI from 5 years ago is reviewed with Tania in the room and does indeed reveal multilevel disc bulges and facet joint arthropathy. Additionally, a small annular tear is identified in the L4–L5 disc.

Assessment and Plan

Having heard Tania's presentation, what does she likely have and what is the next step that you would take as her treating physician?

Tania has obviously been through a lot with her lower back pain. There are many concerning features in Tania's case. First, Tania has had her pain for a long time, has undergone numerous injections, and is still without a diagnosis. Further, one of the most common sources of lower back and buttock pain in her particular case is sacroiliac joint pain and while she did have sacroiliac joint injections, they were apparently performed without image guidance. As such, the injections cannot truly be deemed diagnostic. Further, her facet joint injections did not afford any long-term relief but there is no note of whether they provided short-term relief from the lidocaine or if there was any attempt to use the facet joint injections diagnostically other than to gauge her response to the steroid. The epidural steroid injections did not help Tania but it is not clear what sort of epidurals were performed or what levels were targeted.

One of the potential pitfalls in a case like Tania's is to hear all of the interventional procedures that have been performed and assume that an algorithmic interventional spine approach has not helped her. In fact, it would appear that interventional spine medicine was not optimally applied to Tania and so it is important to step back and consider what is known and what is not known.

Tania has chronic lower back pain without a radicular component. She has a relatively average MRI with mild arthritis and an annular tear at L4–L5. The MRI is 5 years old, and although the symptoms have not largely changed, it is appropriate to get a more up-to-date MRI, particularly if further interventional procedures are planned.

Tania has had multiple failed procedures and is taking opiates to manage her pain. Part of Tania's frustration is that she does not understand why she has the pain and it does not appear that anyone has ever explained to her why different procedures were performed or what might be causing her pain.

The first step to helping Tania is to help her understand and make sense of her pain. By explaining to Tania what is known about chronic lower back pain, and in particular the three most common sources of lower back pain, and by explaining the appropriate steps to arrive at a diagnosis, Tania understands the need for injections and a new MRI. Also, and importantly, rather than being a passive voyager on the receiving end of lots of needles and medications, Tania can begin to feel that she is actively participating in the steps needed to find out what is causing her pain and eliminate the problem. This sense of empowerment is important for Tania, as it is for many people.

After discussing the various options with Tania, it is agreed that she will obtain a new MRI first and then the next steps will be decided.

Follow-Up

Tania went for a new MRI and brought it with her to her follow-up appointment. The repeat MRI is unchanged from her previous MRI. After reviewing the new MRI with Tania, it is agreed to begin the diagnostic process with a diagnostic sacroiliac joint injection. The sacroiliac joint is selected because it is arguably the least invasive diagnostic injection option, her pain started post-pregnancy which suggests sacroiliac joint involvement, and her physical examination was certainly consistent with a sacroiliac joint etiology. Still, it is emphasized to Tania that the sacroiliac joint is a "best first guess" and that even if it turns out to be negative, it is important to learn this so that it can be effectively crossed off the list and the next diagnostic possibility can be pursued.

Tania is taken to the procedure room where a fluoroscopically guided bilateral sacroiliac joint injection is performed using lidocaine for anesthetic and betamethasone for the steroid. Immediately after the injection, Tania is taken back to her room and she is in tears because for the first time in over a decade, she has no pain in her lower back and buttocks. Tania is quite obviously in blissful disbelief to have the pain finally relieved.

Tania is cautioned to realize that her initial pain relief is just the anesthetic and that her pain is not really "gone" yet, but of course this is an encouraging sign. Tania is given a pain diary to rate how much her pain is relieved over the next 8 h.

Tania returns 2 weeks later with her pain diary in hand. Her pain diary revealed 100 % improvement in pain for 2 h, 90 % improvement until 4 h, and then 30 % improvement that lasted for the remaining 4 h when she stopped keeping track. Tania also reports 4 days after the injection, her pain again went away, and at 2 weeks postinjection, she feels about 80–90 % better.

Tania is naturally thrilled with the result of the injection. She has cut her pain medication down to 3 times per day but says she is mostly now taking it out of habit and because she is afraid to stop taking the medication rather than because of the pain. She has not taken a muscle relaxer to help her sleep in 2 weeks. Tania would like to come off of her pain medications completely but is afraid of withdrawal.

Because the pain is so much better at 2 weeks, it is agreed that Tania will slowly taper off of her narcotic medications and start a physical therapy program focused on lumbar stabilization exercises, hip strengthening, and stretching.

Tania returned 3 months later. She had stopped taking her pain medication and had lost 20 lb from working out in the gym. She is thrilled to have her life back. Tania was concerned, however, because the pain in the lower back and buttocks had started to return. The pain was now 60 % better than her baseline, but it was getting slowly worse and was making working out and doing her therapeutic exercises difficult. Because of this, it was agreed that a second sacroiliac joint injection would be performed.

Following the repeat bilateral fluoroscopically guided sacroiliac joint injection, she was again given the pain diary after the injection and again she had complete relief of her pain for 2 h after the injection followed by a slow recurrence of the pain as the lidocaine wore off followed by complete resolution of the pain 4 days later.

Tania returned 2 weeks later to discuss her pain relief and her prognosis. A full discussion was done with Tania regarding the option of radiofrequency rhizotomy of the sacroiliac joints, but because she had been doing so well and because the second sacroiliac joint injection relieved the remaining pain, Tania resumed her home exercise program following the second injection. Fortunately, with the continued exercise, Tania's pain remained abated.

Chapter 24
Clinical Case #6: Frank

Frank is a 68-year-old retired auto worker. He is being referred to this office from his primary care doctor. Frank reports a 20-year history of intermittent lower back pain that got much worse and more constant 2 years ago. He says that 2 years ago, for no apparent reason, he started having worsening lower back and buttock pain that was worse on the right than the left. The pain was mostly dull and aching and was worse when he would go for a walk. A year ago, it got to the point where he was having trouble walking his dog more than a block. At that time, he went to his primary care doctor who sent him to physical therapy.

Frank went to physical therapy and he felt that it was helpful for a while. He would do his stretches in the morning and that seemed to loosen him up so he could take his dog for longer walks. However, about 6 months ago the pain got much worse in his lower back and it began radiating into the right leg. Again he was unable to identify a trigger for the pain getting worse. The pain radiated into the posterior and lateral thigh and into the lower leg to the foot. He had numbness and tingling in the right foot whenever he would stand for more than a few minutes. He tried taking 800 mg of ibuprofen three times a day but it did not help the pain and his stomach started to hurt when he took the medication. He went back to his primary care doctor who told him to take Tylenol three times per day instead of the ibuprofen and sent him back to physical therapy.

This time the physical therapy was not able to help Frank at all. Tylenol did nothing for his pain. Frank reported that his pain limited him from participating with the physical therapy exercises and the passive modalities only made Frank feel better "for a few minutes." Worse, Frank noticed that he was tripping over his feet. He denies any falls but he says that he has almost fallen several times. His primary care doctor then ordered an MRI of the lumbar spine. The MRI revealed a multilevel facet joint arthropathy, a central L4–L5 disc herniation, and an L5–S1 grade I spondylolisthesis and a superimposed right L5–S1 paracentral disc herniation. His primary care doctor then referred Frank to this office.

Frank says that the pain in his lower back is worse than the leg pain. When sitting, the pain is rated as a 2/10 on VAS. When standing for 1 min, the pain in the

G. Cooper, *Non-Operative Treatment of the Lumbar Spine*,
DOI 10.1007/978-3-319-21443-6_24

lower back is 4/10 on VAS. When standing for 10 min or walking a block, the pain is 8/10 and if he continues to stand and/or walk, then the pain will become a 10/10. Bending forward makes the pain better. As the pain gets worse, the numbness in his right foot gets worse. He says that both of his legs feel "a little weak."

Frank reports that he has had increasing trouble with many activities of daily living such as tying his shoes and buttoning his shirts, and he has noticed that his handwriting has gotten much worse in the last couple of months and he has no idea as to why. He says that no one had asked him that previously and he had just figured that he was "getting old."

For the pain, his primary care doctor has recently given him tramadol and he does find that a little helpful and he can function at home on the medication but he is uncomfortable driving while taking it because the tramadol does make him feel a little dizzy. He denies any change in bowel or bladder habits.

Physical Examination

On physical examination, Frank is 5′10″ and 180 lb. He has a muscular build. His gait is wide based and antalgic. He has pain with lumbar extension and he has pain with bilateral oblique lumbar extension that is worse with oblique extension to the right than the left.

Frank has numbness to light touch in the bilateral feet. He has 4+/5 right hip abductor strength, 5−/5 right extensor hallucis longus, and 5−/5 left hip abductor strength. He has a positive straight leg raise on the right at 40° and positive straight leg raise on the left at 60°.

Frank's lumbar paraspinals are diffusely tender but most tender on the right over the L5 and S1 paraspinals. His sacroiliac joints are tender. The right sacroiliac joint reveals greater tenderness than the left. He has a negative FABER test bilaterally. He has a positive Hoffman's test bilaterally and positive Babinski bilaterally. He has 3+ patella and 2+ Achilles reflexes bilaterally.

Assessment and Plan

Having heard Frank's presentation, what does he likely have and what is the next step that you would take as his treating physician?

Frank's history, physical examination, and MRI findings are certainly consistent with lumbar spinal stenosis, likely facet joint pain, and a bilateral, right > left lumbar radiculopathy affecting the L5 nerve roots. However, there are a few findings that are very concerning for another serious medical problem.

Consider Frank's gait. Frank's apparent L5 radiculopathy could explain the pain, numbness, gait antalgia, and weakness in the hip abductors and the extensory hallucis longus. However, in addition to gait problems, Frank has difficulty with fine motor activity in his upper extremities. What explains his increasing difficulty with tasks such as buttoning shirts and what explains his worsening handwriting? To that end, what explains the positive Babinski and Hoffman's sign bilaterally?

Whenever a patient presents with gait antalgia, particularly with worsening gait antalgia, it is important to ask about upper extremity signs of fine motor coordination problems such as manipulating buttons, quality of handwriting, tying shoes, and manipulating small objects. When a patient has any or especially all of those symptoms present, it is concerning for a cervical myelopathy. When a patient has all of those symptoms and also a positive Babinski and Hoffman's sign, it is very concerning for a potential cervical myelopathy.

Cervical myelopathy is not a specifically covered problem in this book, but it is something that is important for the spine physician—or any physician—to keep in the back of her mind as it is too serious to miss. A cervical myelopathy would not cause Frank's pain but it is likely contributing to his gait problems and his upper extremity difficulties.

It is explained to Frank that he clearly has one problem (the lumbar radiculopathy) and he likely has one other (the facet joint pain) and maybe a third problem (the cervical myelopathy). As such, he is scheduled for two things—a bilateral L5 transforaminal epidural steroid injection to address his pain and L5 signs and symptoms and an MRI of the cervical spine to rule out a cervical myelopathy.

Follow-Up

Frank had the lumbar transforaminal epidural steroid injection the next day. He experienced immediate pain relief after the epidural steroid injection. He had his cervical MRI a week later and returned for follow-up evaluation 2 weeks after the epidural steroid injection. Frank was very pleased at his follow-up visit as he noted that 60 % of his pain was gone and his numbness was much improved in his feet. Frank reported being able to walk "a little better" and generally felt "a little more steady" than before. He was also able to tolerate standing for longer than previous.

Unfortunately, Frank's cervical MRI was nothing to celebrate. He had severe central spinal stenosis at C6–7 with cord compression and high intensity signal changes in the spinal cord at that level consistent with myelomalacia.

Frank was seated with his wife and his MRI was reviewed in detail with them both. It was explained why it was important for him to see a spine surgeon even though his back was feeling better.

Because Frank's lower back and legs were feeling so much better, it was agreed to not do anything further with his lumbar spine until he had a chance to talk with a spine surgeon about the possibility of cervical decompressive surgery. Because of the nature of the problem, it was explained to Frank that he needed to act sooner than later to prevent progression of the cord compression which could potentially lead to paralysis.

Frank was told that he should call one of the two surgeons' contact information provided and if he could not be seen within 2 days that he should call the office back so that the visit could be facilitated quicker as this could really not wait. He was told that he should not have anyone manipulate his neck and should be as careful as possible to not have any accidents or falls that could further jeopardize his cervical spine.

Frank was seen by a neurosurgeon the next day and it was recommended that he undergo a decompression and fusion surgery at the C6–7 level. Frank was nervous about the idea of surgery in his cervical spine, particularly because he did not have any neck pain or radiating arm pain and because the surgeon did not even guarantee that his walking would improve or that his upper extremity coordination would improve after the surgery. He was appropriately told he needed the surgery to prevent worsening of the problem and potentially paralysis. Despite the urgency of the problem, Frank ended up getting two more surgical opinions in the next 2 weeks. Both additional consults agreed that decompression and fusion at C6-7 was needed. Frank underwent the surgery on the third week.

Frank returned to the office 5 weeks after his cervical spine surgery. His neck was feeling a little stiff but he was otherwise doing well. Frank was returning to say thanks for recognizing the potential for paralysis from his cervical spine because he now realized how serious his condition had been, and he also returned because the pain in his lower back and leg had been doing much better for a few weeks after the injection but in the last couple of weeks the pain had pretty much returned to baseline.

Of note, Frank reported that his handwriting had not improved after the cervical spine surgery but he did think that it was a little easier to button his clothing. He was optimistic that his fine motor coordination would continue to improve and had some exercises that he had been given to work on that at home.

Now that Frank's cervical spine was stabilized and he had exercises to do for his fine motor coordination, the focus could be turned to the lumbar spine. It was agreed to repeat the bilateral L5 transforaminal epidural steroid injection as this had helped a lot before. This time after the injection, Frank went to physical therapy to focus on gait training, lumbar stabilization and hip stabilization exercises, and hip flexor and knee extensor stretching.

Frank returned 4 weeks after the bilateral L5 transforaminal epidural steroid injection. His lower back and legs were feeling 70 % better. He felt as though the injection got him the 70 % improvement 1 week after the injection but that the physical therapy was not making the pain any better in the last 3 weeks. He did note that he felt stronger overall and he felt that his gait was definitely much improved. Also, his numbness had resolved. While he felt 70 % better, Frank *really* wanted to feel better still.

After a discussion, it was agreed to perform a repeat bilateral L5 transforaminal epidural steroid injection. Frank tolerated the repeat injection very well. After the injection, Frank returned to physical therapy for 3 more weeks. After the 3 weeks, Frank felt he had learned his home exercise program and he continued doing his exercises at home.

Frank returned for follow-up evaluation 6 weeks after the repeat bilateral L5 transforaminal epidural steroid injection. He reported that his pain was 85–90 % improved overall. He was pleased with his progress. He still had pain and discomfort but it was "very livable" and it did not deter him from doing the activities that he enjoyed.

Also importantly, Frank reported being much more steady on his feet. His gait had returned to close to normal and he felt like he was "more or less" back to his "old self." Frank understood the importance of continuing his home exercise regimen and he did just that.

Of note, it is possible that another epidural steroid injection would have relieved the remaining 10–15 % of the person's pain. It is also possible that the remaining pain was from the facet joints and he may have done well with a facet joint injection or ultimately a radiofrequency rhizotomy. However, Frank was feeling so good after the injections and physical therapy that doing more from an interventional standpoint would inherently have seen diminished returns (since most of the pain was gone anyway) and since Frank was not particularly bothered by his remaining pain, what purpose would those further injections have served?

For Frank, after discussing the relative pros and cons of another injection, it seemed the better course was to emphasize the importance of continuing his home exercises and see where things went from there. As it turns out, Frank returned a year and a half later with his wife who was having lower back pain. For Frank's part, he was still feeling about 80 % better, doing his exercises, and feeling good about his quality of life. He also mentioned that his handwriting had never returned to "normal" but it was much improved from before the cervical spine surgery.

Chapter 25
Clinical Case #7: Natasha

Natasha is a 42-year-old homemaker and mother of three children, ages 12, 8, and 4. She presents with an 11-month history of lower back pain. Natasha is being referred to this office by her primary care doctor. Natasha's pain does not radiate into the legs. She denies any numbness, tingling, or burning in the legs. The legs do not feel weak. The pain is described as "sharp" and is centralized around the L5–S1 level. The pain is worse with sitting. She says that going for long car rides is "very difficult" because the pain becomes extremely intense. Standing and walking around makes the pain better. In general, she feels that the more she moves, the better she tends to feel unless she does "too much."

Natasha rates the pain as 5/10 on average on VAS. She says that she had to go on a 2 h car ride a couple of weeks ago and the pain was 9/10 on VAS by the end of the ride, and for the next few hours afterward the pain continued to be "at least an 8/10."

Natasha says that at times the pain is only 2–3/10. Her lower back is generally more stiff and aching in the morning. As she gets moving, the pain is better, but then anytime she sits for more than a few minutes, the pain is back to a 6 or 7/10 on VAS. Lifting her 4-year-old son is very painful for her. Any activity where she has to bend forward and pick something up is painful unless she is very careful with her lifting posture.

Natasha has been to her friend who is a massage therapist and she says that massages definitely make the pain better for a few hours but then the pain always returns. She has not taken any pain medication because she does not want to "just mask" the pain with medications. She has not had any imaging studies. She has not been to physical therapy. Natasha says that she used to work out on a regular basis and take lots of different types of cardio classes but she has not done that in several years because she has been so busy with her three children.

Other than her lower back pain, Natasha is in very good general health. She has seasonal allergies and she has a history of a tonsillectomy. She does not take any medications on a regular basis.

G. Cooper, *Non-Operative Treatment of the Lumbar Spine*,
DOI 10.1007/978-3-319-21443-6_25

Physical Examination

On physical examination, Natasha is 5′6″ and 125 lb and appears generally fit and in good health. Her gait is normal. She has pain with trunk flexion that is most notable at 30°. She has no pain with lumbar extension or bilateral lumbar oblique extension. Her strength is 5/5 in the lower extremities bilaterally. Her sensation is intact in the lower extremities bilaterally. She has a negative straight leg raise bilaterally. She has a negative slump test bilaterally.

Natasha's lumbar paraspinals are diffusely tender but the tenderness is most pronounced over the bilateral L5 and S1 paraspinals. Natasha's sacroiliac joints are mildly tender bilaterally. She has a negative FABER test bilaterally. She has brisk and symmetric patella and Achilles reflexes. She has full, pain-free range of motion of her bilateral hips. She has good overall flexibility in her knee extensors and hip flexors. She has negative Babinski and Hoffman's reflexes bilaterally.

Assessment and Plan

Having heard Natasha's presentation, what does she likely have and what is the next step that you would take as her treating physician?

Natasha has chronic lower back pain that clinically is most consistent with discogenic lower back pain. In fact, it may be said that she presents with a classic case of discogenic lower back pain. Her pain is axial, flexion biased, and worse in the morning.

While clinically Natasha seems to clearly have discogenic lower back pain, it must be remembered that from an evidence-based perspective, her chance of having discogenic lower back pain is around 40 % versus facet joint pain (15 %), sacroiliac joint pain (10–15 %), and other sources (30–35 %). Therefore, it may be said that clinically she appears to have discogenic lower back pain, whereas academically she most likely does not.

Natasha is very interested in the pathophysiology of her problem. The mechanics of her spine are explained to her as are the different potential offending pathophysiologies. Regardless of the underlying pathophysiology, she understands that her relative deconditioning over the past several years has likely contributed to her current problem. Natasha does not like medications and is not interested in any "quick fixes." She likes the idea of physical therapy as a beginning point in her treatment and is very motivated to get started. As such, she is prescribed a 6-week course of physical therapy with a focus on extension-biased lumbar stabilization exercises.

Follow-Up

Natasha returns 7 weeks later. She has been doing physical therapy for over a month. She reports that she enjoys the physical therapy and feels stronger overall. Her pain is "about 30 % better." She is frustrated that her pain is persistent despite her work in therapy. Given the chronicity of her pain, it is decided that she should obtain imaging studies of her spine.

When considering what imaging studies to order, it is helpful to consider the relative merits. X-rays would rule out a spondylolisthesis, fracture, and certain other bony pathologies such as facet joint arthropathy but X-rays would still not negate the need for an MRI which would show those same problems and more. Additionally, X-rays would entail radiation and MRI entails none. CT scan would reveal bony pathology as well as soft tissue pathologies, but CT scans entail a very significant amount of radiation and still don't detail the soft tissue as well as an MRI.

As such, an MRI of the lumbosacral spine is obtained. Even before the MRI is ordered, it is explained to Natasha that the MRI is almost certainly not going to be diagnostic of her pain. MRIs fail to identify most annular tears in the lumbar spine and even when an annular tear is present, it may be asymptomatic. Facet joint arthropathy is very common in asymptomatic people even at the age of 42 and so is not particularly interesting when found. The MRI is obtained as a piece of the puzzle and an important piece, but in her case of axial lower back pain in the absence of neurologic findings, the MRI is obtained chiefly to rule out very unusual problems, to provide peace of mind, and to allow for interventional spinal procedures to be performed should they be deemed necessary.

The MRI of the lumbosacral spine is obtained and reveals mild facet joint arthropathy at L5–S1 bilaterally and an annular tear at L5–S1. Otherwise, the study is normal. The results of the MRI are reviewed with Natasha. As previously mentioned, the presence of facet joint arthropathy is not surprising as it is a relatively ubiquitous finding (recall that about 50 % of 30-year-old people have arthritis in their spine.) The annular tear at L5–S1 is certainly consistent with the diagnosis of discogenic lower back pain but as mentioned some people do have asymptomatic annular tears so the diagnosis is still not certain.

Natasha is somewhat relieved that the MRI is within the normal range of wear and tear for her age. She is feeling 30 % better from the first 6 weeks of physical therapy and would like to continue with therapy before considering an injection to see if she continues to improve. She returns to physical therapy for another 4 weeks. After a month, she returns for a follow-up visit.

At Natasha's follow-up visit, she reports that she is feeling 50 % improved. She has been discharged from physical therapy because she knows all of her exercises and can perform them on her own. She does them for about 20 min every night. She is feeling good enough that she wants to continue with her exercises before doing anything else. She asks if there is anything else she could do on her own to help expedite her recovery. She has said that she misses working out in the gym and asks if she can return to exercise classes. She asks specifically about running and if that is bad for her back.

In addition to her home exercise program from physical therapy, Natasha is advised to join a Pilates class for enhanced core strengthening and flexibility. Additionally, exercise in general is encouraged. The general rules for exercise in a person like Natasha include that she has not exercised in a long time so she should remember to start gradually. It didn't take a week for Natasha to get out of shape and so she should not expect to get back into shape in a week either. She is making lifestyle changes for the long haul and the changes should be slow, steady, and consistent. Natasha is reminded to start slow and build up with both the intensity of her exercise routines as well as their duration.

The second rule for Natasha with exercise is that she needs to listen to her body. If she is doing an exercise and it is creating pain in her lower back then she should back off of that particular exercise and find another exercise. Movement is great for the spine and for joints in general. The proverb for joints is that if you don't use them, you lose them, and the same may be said to be generally true about spines. The human spine craves movement. But that movement should not be painful and so if pain is being created, then another movement should be substituted. If using an elliptical machine creates pain for Natasha, for example, then she should stop using the elliptical and find another exercise. After a few weeks, she may return to the elliptical and see if she is able to use it without pain. If it still causes pain, she should again find a different exercise.

When thinking of pain with movement, it is important to distinguish spinal pain from muscular pain. Natasha has not worked out in a long time and so it is to be expected (and even a little welcomed) that she should have some muscular pain as she uses and pushes muscles that she has not used (or perhaps felt) in many years. It is important, therefore, that Natasha be able to identify the difference between spinal pain and muscular pain because if she stopped every time her muscles felt sore, then she would truly have a hard time progressing her routine. If Natasha is having a hard time distinguishing the different types of pain, then it is important that she discuss it with her doctor or physical therapist.

The question of running and lower back pain is a very common one and a much disputed one at that. There are three different fields of thought. The first field of thought is that running is bad for the lower back and should be avoided because of the constant pounding of the activity. The thinking goes that the repetitive impact caused by running creates stress through the spine and this causes an accelerated wear and tear cascade through the spine that should be avoided in anyone with lower back problems. While it is true that stress and wear and tear may be created in the spine by running, it is not true that this has been shown to be causally related to lower back pain. Therefore, the causation of running and increased wear and tear in the spine remains informed conjecture.

The second field of thought regarding running and lower back pain is that the repetitive impact of running is good for the lumbar spine because the impact on the spine compresses the disc, forcing the disc to achieve better vascular flow and therefore better nutrition and this results in a healthier overall spine. There is some conceptual value to this thought process but again no hard data to support the thought that running is causally related to reduced incidence of lower back pain. There is of course value to overall exercise decreasing morbidity and maintaining a healthier weight and this has positive relation to reduced lower back pain. However, to the question of whether or not running in particular is good for reducing lower back pain and spinal problems in general, there is no hard data to rely on.

The third field of thought, and the one subscribed to by this author and also by Natasha's doctor, is that it depends on the individual and the individual's circumstance. If running makes Natasha feel great, then Natasha should run. If running makes Natasha's back hurt, then Natasha should find a different sport. If running were Natasha's only and most cherished athletic outlet (it isn't) and it also caused her back pain (it didn't), then it would be important for Natasha to cross-train to strengthen her other muscles so that running would no longer cause pain so that she could participate with running, realizing that it might not be the best sport for her given that it tends to increase her pain at times.

For Natasha, she continued her physical therapy home exercises, started a Pilates class, and decided to not chance it with running and instead started taking different cardio dance classes at the gym. She reported back 2 months later that she was feeling great and was pain-free.

A definitive diagnosis was never found for Natasha because she improved without the need for diagnostic injections. In summary, Natasha likely had discogenic lower back pain that was brought on or worsened by a gradual deconditioning of her muscles and overall strength. Natasha recognized this and put in the work to reverse the muscular imbalances and problems. As she did this, the biomechanical stress on her back was reduced and in turn the pain slowly and gradually improved. Over time, Natasha integrated her physical therapy home exercises with her Pilates into her own unique workout regimen that she enjoyed and fit her lifestyle. Because she was able to do that, when she returned to the office a year later with her husband for *his* lower back pain, she was happy to report that she was still pain-free.

Chapter 26
Clinical Case #8: Jack

Jack is a 78-year-old retired salesman who presents with a 3-week history of left lower back pain that began without any identifiable inciting cause. Jack has a past medical history that includes coronary artery disease with two stents placed, hypertension, diabetes type II, benign prostate hypertrophy, chronic obstructive pulmonary disease, gall bladder surgery, and diverticulitis. Although his medical history is significant, Jack considers himself to be "pretty healthy all things considered."

Jack enjoys playing golf and until 3 weeks ago was able to walk 18 holes of the golf course. Jack says that he does not "work out" but he stays active. In addition to golf, Jack occasionally goes bowling and he also goes on frequent long walks with his wife. One of Jack and his wife's favorite activities is to spend an afternoon walking through a museum.

The pain in Jack's left lower back is sharp in character. He says that the pain is 9/10 on VAS at worst and 4/10 at best. The pain does not radiate into the lower extremity. The pain is worse with prolonged standing. Twisting makes the pain much worse. Sitting is generally better than standing, but if he sits for more than 20 min, then the pain becomes worse again. Jack is very frustrated because he does not understand where the pain came from. Multiple times while talking in the office, Jack says "but I just don't get it because I didn't do anything" to cause the pain.

Jack has mild numbness in the bilateral feet that he says has been there for years and he says that he has been told that the numbness is from his diabetes. He does not feel weak in the legs. He went to a chiropractor a week ago and he felt better after being treated but then the pain "came right back a couple of hours later" and his primary care doctor told him to come to this office. Jack has tried taking Tylenol for the pain and says it helps "a little." Jack has taken Aleve and finds that to be "pretty good" for the pain. Over the last 3 weeks, Jack notes that the pain has not gotten much better or gotten much worse.

For his multiple medical conditions, Jack takes many medications including Plavix for his CAD and stents. He denies any change in bowel or bladder habits. He notes that he has had back pain intermittently in the past but it has never been anywhere near this bad before or lasted this long.

G. Cooper, *Non-Operative Treatment of the Lumbar Spine*,
DOI 10.1007/978-3-319-21443-6_26

Physical Examination

On physical examination, Jack is 5′9″ and 170 lb. He has a thin but muscular build. Jack exhibits some mild thoracic hyperkyphosis. He has a normal gait but he is in obvious pain when he transitions from sit to stand or from stand to sit. Jack has pain with lumbar flexion as well as lumbar extension. He has severe pain with left lumbar oblique extension but no pain with right lumbar oblique extension. He has very significant tenderness in the left lumbar paraspinals and his left quadratus lumborum muscle is particularly tender although no trigger point with a referral pain pattern is identified. His sacroiliac joints are not tender. Jack has a negative straight leg raise bilaterally and negative slump test bilaterally.

Jack has 5/5 strength in his lower extremities bilaterally. He has intact sensation to light touch except mildly decreased sensation in the bilateral feet. He has no reflexes in the patella or Achilles reflexes bilaterally. His hips have restricted range of motion bilaterally but range of motion does not produce pain. Jack's hip flexors and knee extensors are very tight to passive range of motion testing.

Assessment and Plan

Having heard Jack's presentation, what does he likely have and what is the next step that you would take as his treating physician?

Jack has acute left lower back pain. With his age and comorbidities, it is perhaps tempting to consider this as a more significant problem than it may in fact be. The pain has only been present for 3 weeks and prior to the pain, which began without inciting event, Jack was playing golf and leading a very active lifestyle. It is very possible, and in fact probable, that Jack has a muscle strain in his left lower back, likely in his left quadratus lumborum.

Jack's concern that he "didn't do anything" to cause his pain is a very common one. Often, an inciting event—even when the cause is a muscle spasm—cannot be identified. This is particularly true in the geriatric population. A helpful way to conceptualize this, particularly for patients, is to recognize that as we all get older, our bodies experience more "wear and tear," and the spine develops arthritis. Recall in fact that by 60 years of age, 100% of people will have arthritis in their spine. While that arthritis may indeed never cause *any* symptoms, it is also reasonable to suppose that the arthritic changes *may* predispose to a greater propensity to develop muscle spasms and various other aches and pains with less provocation than it would have taken to cause a spasm when that same person was, say, 20 years of age.

The pain that Jack is experiencing is severe and must be addressed promptly. Indeed, there is a concern for Jack that given his age and comorbidities, if he were to spend too much time lying on his couch because of the pain, then when the pain is gone, it may be that much more difficult for him to get back off his couch. While anyone who spends a month lying in bed will need a long time to rehabilitate themselves to get stronger and back to themselves, this is particularly true in people who are older and sicker. A decent rule of thumb is that for every day a person spends lying in bed, it takes 2 days to build back that strength once out of bed.

For Jack, the best approach at the time of his presentation is to treat the problem as a muscle spasm. Jack liked going to his chiropractor and would like to go back assuming no contraindications. Jack's findings were reviewed with him and his wife. It was agreed that Jack would return to his chiropractor and also go to physical therapy. One of the problems that Jack has is that he is very active, but he has not been doing anything to make himself stronger or more flexible so that he would be less likely to develop injuries such as the current one.

One of the goals of physical therapy for Jack is to help get the pain to go away. Along with the chiropractor, the physical therapist may use soft tissue mobilization, ultrasound, and electrical stimulation to help with the muscle spasm. However, the other goal of physical therapy is to give Jack a set of exercises that he can use once the pain is gone to perform on a regular basis to make it less likely that the pain returns in the future. For Jack, this will mean strengthening his lumbar stabilizing muscles and stretching his hips, hip flexors, and knee extensor muscles.

Jack at first protests the need for continued physical therapy exercises because he is "so active." This is a common resistance among people who are active. It is explained to Jack that his activity is great for a variety of reasons including improving his cardiovascular health, mental health, pulmonary health, and strength and for his general well-being. However, in a similar way to the point that you would not send a professional athlete out to his sport without cross-training him first so that it is less likely that he would get injured, it is important that Jack cross-train himself so that when he goes out and plays golf and goes for long walks, it is less likely that he gets injured.

Another important point for Jack is that he needs to stop taking his Aleve. Aleve, like other NSAIDs, increases the risk of bleeding into the gastrointestinal system. With Jack taking Plavix, this risk is even greater. NSAIDs and Plavix are contraindicated together and should be avoided. Jack was advised to continue with his Tylenol and also was prescribed a specialty compound cream consisting of a muscle relaxer and lidocaine.

Follow-Up

Jack received his compound pain cream and went to chiropractic care and physical therapy for 4 weeks. At his follow-up visit, Jack reported that the pain in his lower back was much better at first with the cream. Over the last 2 weeks, he has not needed the cream because the pain was completely gone and he had been able to return to his full activities of daily living including playing golf. Jack reported that he was doing "some of the exercises" that he had learned at physical therapy at home. He was also continuing to see the chiropractor once per week because he felt that it kept him feeling looser and more mobile.

It was emphasized to Jack that he should continue with his exercises to make the chance of re-injury less likely. At the same time, it was emphasized to Jack that if he did develop lower back pain again, he should not hesitate to call.

Something to keep in mind that many spine specialists have noticed and commented on is that patients are sometimes reluctant to call when pain returns if they have not been doing their exercises. One patient, who was also interestingly a doctor, told this author that he had not called for a follow-up because he felt "guilty" because he had not been doing his exercises and so he felt that the recurrence of pain was at least partially his "fault."

In that particular case, because the patient was also a cardiologist, I told him that this sounded to me equivalent to a patient not calling him with chest pain because he felt guilty that he had not changed his diet and so he felt that he should just deal with the chest pain on his own! Of course, this would be ridiculous and likewise it should be ridiculous for a patient to not call his spine specialist about his lower back pain because he had failed to do his home exercise regimen.

Since that time, I have been careful to point out to my patients that I want to empower them to know how to stay healthy and pain-free. To that end, I want them to know their exercises and understand why they are important for their particular situation. However, it is my job as their doctor to always look out for their best interests no matter what they choose to do. That is to say that if they make an informed decision to not do their exercise for whatever reason, my job is of course to still help them no matter what. Some of my colleagues I know have run into the same issue and so it is always worth reinforcing that our role as healthcare providers is to carry out our fiduciary responsibility to help our patients at every step of the way and counsel good choices but help them even if they choose choices that are less good ones.

Chapter 27
Clinical Case #9: Esther

Esther is a 72-year-old mother of four children and grandmother of eight who presents with a 3-week history of right lower back pain. She says that she has had intermittent right-sided lower back pain for many years, but the pain has always been mild and it had not been bothering her at all for a few months until 3 weeks ago. Three weeks ago, the pain began after taking care of her 6-month-old granddaughter. Esther says that she was lifting her granddaughter a lot on that day and felt the pain in her right lower back but kept lifting her anyway. That night, the pain in the right lower back was "pretty bad" and in the morning she had trouble getting out of bed because of the pain.

The pain in the right lower back does not radiate into the leg. She denies any numbness, tingling, or burning in the leg. The right leg does not feel weak. She rested for the first day when the pain was bad but by the second day, the pain was still "really bad" and she called her primary care doctor.

Her primary care doctor prescribed Naprosyn 500 mg twice a day and a muscle relaxer. Esther took the muscle relaxer but it made her very dizzy so she stopped taking it. The Naprosyn did not seem to help so she called her primary care doctor back the next day. At that point, her primary care doctor prescribed tramadol and told her to rest. Tramadol helped the pain a little and the pain seemed to ease up over the next week.

For the last 2 weeks, she describes the pain as 5/10 on VAS on average. The pain is worse with standing, walking, and twisting. The pain is better with resting. She has not had any imaging studies. She has not been to physical therapy or a chiropractor. The pain woke her up from sleep for the first week but in the last 2 weeks she has not been waking up with the pain. She takes tramadol 3 times a day and feels that this helps her pain significantly. She has continued to take the Naprosyn 500 mg PO twice per day although she does not know if this is helping. She denies any change in bowel or bladder and has not noticed any gait problems other than the pain while walking.

Esther is generally in good medical health. She has a history of high blood pressure and high cholesterol that are both controlled with medication and diet. She has

G. Cooper, *Non-Operative Treatment of the Lumbar Spine*,
DOI 10.1007/978-3-319-21443-6_27

a history of bilateral total knee replacements 4 years ago and the knees have been doing well since then. She does not exercise on a regular basis but she does enjoy walking, doing chores around her house, and taking care of her eight grandchildren. She feels that she is generally a healthy and active person.

Physical Examination

On physical examination, Esther is 5′2″ and 120 lb. She has a cervical anterior carry and thoracic hyperkyphosis. She has a normal gait. With transitions from sit to stand and stand to sit, she has obvious pain in her lower back. She has full lumbar flexion but has pain and restricted range of motion with lumbar extension and she has severe pain with right lumbar oblique extension and mild discomfort with left lumbar oblique extension.

Esther has very significant tenderness in the right lumbar paraspinals and in her right quadratus lumborum muscle in particular. Her right sacroiliac joint is tender. She has a negative straight leg raise bilaterally and negative slump test bilaterally.

Esther has 5/5 strength in her lower extremities bilaterally except 4+/5 bilateral hip abductor strength. She has intact sensation to light touch in her lower extremities. She has brisk and symmetric reflexes in her patella and Achilles. She has negative Babinski and Hoffman's reflexes bilaterally.

Esther's hips have restricted range of motion bilaterally but passive range of motion does not reproduce her pain. Her hip flexors and knee extensors are very tight to passive range of motion testing.

Assessment and Plan

Having heard Esther's presentation, what does she likely have and what is the next step that you would take as her treating physician?

Esther is in good general health and has 3 weeks of right lower back pain. While she may have a number of different pathophysiologies, at the moment all signs point to acute lower back pain caused by a muscle strain likely superimposed on underlying degenerative changes. The tramadol seems to be helping her manage her symptoms. Esther's symptoms improved initially but have been relatively stable over the last 2 weeks.

After a discussion of the different options, it is agreed that Esther will begin physical therapy to focus on passive modalities such as soft tissue mobilization, ultrasound, and electrical stimulation as well as stretching and strengthening exercises to specifically focus on lumbar stabilization exercises, hip abductor strengthening, and hip flexor and knee extensor stretching. It is explained to Esther that it is important to not just get this pain to go away, which will likely happen anyway with a little more time given the acute nature of it and the natural history of acute lower back pain in general. However, in addition to making the pain go away, it is important for Esther to also learn a set of exercises that will make it less likely that she has these kinds of problems in the future.

Esther understands and is excited about the plan. In addition, her Naprosyn is discontinued as she does not believe it is really helping her and instead she starts Duexis (800 mg ibuprofen/26.6 famotidine) TID and is also given a compound cream consisting of cyclobenzaprine and baclofen to help with the muscle spasms.

Follow-Up

Esther returns 4 weeks later and reports that her pain is about 50 % improved. She has continued to take the tramadol and Duexis as well as to use the compound muscle relaxer cream. She is going to physical therapy and particularly enjoys the soft tissue mobilization and ultrasound treatments. She does the exercises but says that she is not sure they are helping her. She does feel a little stronger and overall more stable on her feet than before.

Esther's physical examination is similar to her previous examinations except that now she has less tenderness in her paraspinals and her quadratus lumborum is not particularly tender. Esther is pleased with her improvement and would like to continue with the current plan. Given her improvement, this seems reasonable and so she returns to physical therapy and is instructed to only take the Duexis and tramadol when she has the pain rather than just taking it around the clock at the scheduled intervals as she has been doing.

Esther returns for a follow-up visit in 4 weeks. She reports that she has become frustrated. The pain had seemed like it was getting so much better in the beginning of physical therapy but in the last 4 weeks the pain has changed somewhat and is not getting better. The pain still "feels the same and maybe a little worse" and is localized over the right L4, L5, and S1 region.

Esther reports that she no longer gets the pain when she is sitting. In fact, she is concerned because sitting feels so good that that is all she wants to do. Standing from a sitting position also does not produce much pain. However, standing for any length of time (e.g., greater than 2 min) makes the pain worse. She cannot tolerate standing for more than 20 min before the pain makes her want to sit down. The pain still does not radiate into the legs. She continues to have a lack of any neurologic symptoms in the legs. She has continued to take the Duexis and tramadol and she has continued to use the compound cream. She feels as though all of this is helping but she realizes that at this point the medications are just helping to mask the pain.

On repeat physical examination, Esther has pain with right lumbar oblique extension. She has tenderness over the right lumbar paraspinals as well as over the right sacroiliac joint. However, the tenderness is not as pronounced as on previous examination. She has a negative FABER test, negative straight leg raise, and negative slump test bilaterally. Her gait is non-antalgic. Her strength in the lower extremities is now 5/5 bilaterally including in the hip abductors. Her sensation is intact in the lower extremities and she has brisk and symmetric patella and Achilles reflexes. She has negative Babinski and Hoffman's reflexes bilaterally.

Esther has now had her pain in the right lower back for 1 week shy of 3 months. Given her age and the chronicity of her right axial lower back pain and her lack of response to 8 weeks of physical therapy, it is agreed to order an MRI of the lumbosacral spine.

Esther goes for the MRI and returns for a follow-up visit. The MRI reveals a grade I L2–L3 spondylolisthesis, a multilevel bilateral facet joint arthropathy, an L4–L5 disc bulge, and a multilevel degenerative disc disease that is most severe at L4–L5 and L5–S1.

The results of the MRI are discussed with Esther in the context of her symptoms. At this point, her symptoms are chronic. Her MRI findings are relatively nonspecific which was largely to be expected. Clinically, her signs and symptoms all point to extension-biased right axial chronic lower back pain that is most in line with right-sided facet joint arthropathy causing her pain.

While clinically she appears to have facet joint pain, academically it must be remembered that she has a 40 % chance that her pain is coming from her disc, 30 % that it is coming from her facet joints, 10–15 % that it is coming from her sacroiliac joint, and 10–15 % chance that it is coming from a different pathology.

At this point, it is recommended to Esther that she undergo a diagnostic and potentially therapeutic block of her right L3–L4, L4–L5, and L5–S1 facet joints. Esther is nervous about any spinal injections and asks if there is a downside to waiting. She asks in particular if she could try another round of physical therapy and if there is anything else that has a chance of working. It is explained to Esther that there is no downside to waiting on a potential injection. Her pain is troubling in its own right but it is not "dangerous" per se. There is no perceivable medical downside to continued physical therapy although it has not been helpful over the last 4 weeks.

A real world downside is that Esther has Medicare and Medicare only pays for a certain dollar amount of physical therapy in a year time period. As it happens, Esther was being treated at this point in April and so it was early in the year to use up all of her physical therapy. If she were to use up all her therapy early in the year and then needed the therapy later in the calendar year for an unrelated problem, she may have trouble getting it covered (although she would always have the option of paying out of pocket for it). A reason to persist in physical therapy is that this helps normalize and optimize the biomechanics and prevent any compensatory alterations/adaptations which could produce a domino-like effect in adjacent joints and connective soft tissue potentially resulting in other musculoskeletal problems.

Esther was not concerned about using her physical therapy up as she was fortunate to have the resources to pay for physical therapy out of pocket in the future if it came to that. As to the question of other potential therapeutic options, chiropractic care and acupuncture were both discussed with Esther. She understood the lack of data behind the two approaches but was interested in doing everything she could to get better to see if she could avoid any injections. As such, she elected to go to both acupuncture and chiropractic care as well as another round of physical therapy.

The one medical downside of the plan was her continued use of the medications and of Duexis in particular. As the medications were not helping the problem to go away, she agreed to discontinue the oral medications and just use the muscle relaxing cream for the pain. She also elected to try Tylenol as needed for the pain.

Esther returned 6 weeks later. She reported that she did not feel the acupuncture was helping so after 3 weeks she had decided to stop going to that. She liked going to the chiropractor but only felt that it helped for the day that she was there and sometimes for the next day as well. She had continued as well with the physical therapy and felt that it was helpful and she continued to feel stronger and looser, which she appreciated, but overall she said that despite all of this, the pain was largely unchanged since the last time that she had come to the office.

The bottom line for Esther was that she still could only stand for about 10 min before the pain got "really bad" and by 20 min the pain compelled her to sit down. Tylenol didn't help. She still had some tramadol at home but elected not to take it because she said that if she really wanted the pain to go away all she had to do was sit down. She was particularly disturbed because the pain made it difficult for her to take care of her grandchildren.

Given the persistence of the pain, the lack of response to conservative measures, and the way the pain was negatively impacting her quality of life, it was elected to perform a fluoroscopically guided diagnostic and hopefully therapeutic intra-articular facet joint injection using 4 cm^3 of 1 % lidocaine and 12 mg of Celestone divided evenly between the right L3–L4, L4–L5, and L5–S1 levels.

Esther tolerated the facet joint injection well and there were no complications. After the injection, Esther was given a pain diary to keep for the rest of the day. Esther returned in 2 weeks for a follow-up visit and reviewed her pain diary. At 1 min after the injection, she reported 80 % improvement in pain. At 20 min, she reported 100 % pain relief. The pain relief remained 100 % until hour 4 at which point the pain slowly recurred so that at hour 7 the pain was back to baseline.

When pressed further on her pain diary, Esther was pleased to report that for the first 4 h, Esther was able to stand for as long as she wanted to with absolutely no pain. This was the first time in more than 4 months that Esther could do that and she was very excited about it. Unfortunately, after the lidocaine wore off, the pain returned. Four days after the injection, the pain got "about 30 % better" but that only lasted for 3 days and then the pain returned completely to baseline.

Given Esther's very good diagnostic response to the lidocaine and very poor therapeutic response to the steroid, it was elected to perform a diagnostic medial branch block injection procedure with the intention that if it confirmed facet joint pain, she would undergo a radiofrequency rhizotomy procedure.

Esther underwent medial branch blocks of the right L3–L4, L4–L5, and L5–S1 facet joints using 2 % lidocaine and again had nearly 100 % pain relief for 4 h followed by a rapid recurrence of pain so that at 7 h, her pain was back to baseline. Again during the 100 % pain relief, she was able to stand unrestricted with no pain for as long as she wanted.

The pros and cons of a third diagnostic injection repeating the medial branch blocks was discussed. On the one hand, it would make the diagnosis more certain given that the first injection was an intra-articular injection and therefore may carry less clear diagnostic weight. On the other hand, both diagnostic blocks of the facet joint were positive and not only did she receive pain relief but she was able to functionally stand unrestricted during her pain relief (which anecdotally may seem less likely than if the pain relief were purely placebo driven). Given all of the above, it was agreed that she would proceed with the radiofrequency rhizotomy procedure.

Esther had the rhizotomy procedure the following week and returned for follow-up 3 weeks later. At follow-up visit, Esther reported that she had been sore for about a week after the rhizotomy procedure but then about two and a half weeks after the procedure, the pain virtually went away in the right lower back. To Esther, it felt like a miracle. She was able to stand and walk again without pain.

Although Esther's pain was gone, it was explained to her again that the nerves tend to regenerate within 6–18 months and that the pain may return if that were to happen. Ideally, Esther would use her time when she was feeling better to continue with her lumbar stabilization exercises, hip abductor strengthening, and hip flexor and knee extensor stretching exercises. In addition to helping make it less likely that her facet joint pain would recur, the exercises would be good in general to help prevent future injury to her spine and her hips. Esther understood all of this and said that she would certainly continue with her exercises.

Esther returned 10 months later for a follow-up visit. She reported that over the last 4 weeks, the pain in the right lower back had been returning and slowly getting worse. She said that the pain felt exactly as it had prior to the radiofrequency rhizotomy procedure. The pain was worse with standing and walking and went away completely when she sat down. The pain was limiting her to the point where she could stand about a half hour before she had to sit down. Every week, she said, the pain was getting worse and her standing tolerance was also getting worse.

Esther reported that she had indeed continued to do her physical therapy exercises for the last 10 months. She spent 20–30 min every day doing her exercises. She felt stronger and more flexible overall. She said that she did not regret doing the exercises even though her pain had returned because she feels that she is more stable on her feet and less likely to get injured overall.

At follow-up, Esther asked if she could have the radiofrequency rhizotomy procedure repeated for the pain but says that she will continue with her home exercises into the future and hopefully the next time the pain will not return.

It was discussed with Esther that she could return to physical therapy, chiropractic, and/or acupuncture but Esther preferred to have the rhizotomy procedure repeated. Given that the symptoms were unchanged from before and her physical examination was not changed (except improved flexibility and strength), repeated diagnostic facet joint blocks were not needed and the repeat radiofrequency rhizotomy procedure was performed. Again, Esther had a great response to the procedure and was pain-free at 3 weeks follow-up.

Reflecting on Esther's case, there are a couple of points worth highlighting. In the beginning, she presented with acute lower back pain. While it is true that in the end her pain turned out to be facet joint based, it would not have been appropriate to inject her facet joints at that time given the acute nature of the pain. At her first presentation, there was simply no way of knowing that her pain would turn out to be anything other than a muscle spasm.

Esther's MRI is also worth noting. Esther had a spondylolisthesis at L2–L3. This spondylolisthesis could have been causing her pain but it was higher than her pain and epidemiologically much less likely than her facet joints, discs, and sacroiliac joints to be the source of her pain. It was right to ignore the spondylolisthesis and interrogate the lower facet joints that were more likely to have been causing her pain. If the pain had persisted despite the facet joint injections, despite the sacroiliac joint injections, and despite a transforaminal epidural steroid injection, then considering the L2–L3 spondylolisthesis as a potential source of her pain would have been appropriate at that time.

Chapter 28
Clinical Case #10: Rebecca

Rebecca is a 34-year-old attorney and a mother of two who presents with an 18-month history of right lower back pain, buttock pain, and right lower extremity pain. The pain began insidiously without any specific identifiable inciting event 18 months ago when her youngest son was 2 years old. At first the pain she reports that the pain was mild. She tried to "just ignore the pain." She initially attributed the pain to taking care of her kids, including lifting her 2-year-old son into and out of the car, working long hours, and generally not taking better care of herself. However, over following 3 months her pain gradually worsened to the point that she realized it was affecting her work performance and making it difficult for her to take care of her children. At that point, she went to see her primary care physician who sent her to a pain management doctor.

The pain management doctor that Rebecca initially went to immediately ordered an MRI of her lumbar spine. The MRI revealed a small right L5–S1 disc bulge and she was diagnosed with a right L5 and S1 radiculopathy. She was given an L5–S1 interlaminar epidural steroid injection and sent to physical therapy. Unfortunately, the interlaminar epidural steroid injection did not help at all. She went to physical therapy and that did not help her pain either.

She returned to the first pain management doctor after 3 weeks of physical therapy and had a repeat L5–S1 interlaminar epidural steroid injection. Again, the injection did not help and two more weeks of physical therapy did not help either. When asked what was done during her physical therapy sessions, Rebecca reports frequent treatments of hot packs, massage, and extension-based stretches.

Rebecca became frustrated with the first pain management doctor and also with physical therapy. She then went to a chiropractor on the recommendation of a friend. She saw the chiropractor 3 times per week for 3 weeks but the pain did not improve. She returned to the first pain management doctor at that time who in turn gave her a referral to a spine surgeon. Rebecca went to the spine surgeon who told her that he could not help her and she should return to her pain management doctor.

At that time, Rebecca went to a different pain management doctor. That pain management doctor gave her trigger point injections in her lower back and buttock.

G. Cooper, *Non-Operative Treatment of the Lumbar Spine*,
DOI 10.1007/978-3-319-21443-6_28

After the trigger point injections, Rebecca's pain got better for about 3 days but then the pain returned to baseline. She had two more rounds of trigger point injections over the next month and each time she experienced only 2–3 days of partial pain relief.

The pain that Rebecca gets is a sharp pain in her right lower back and buttock. She has right leg pain that she feels is referred from her lower back and buttock but she does not describe it as "sharp" or "shooting" or "electric." Rather, the pain is a vague aching sensation that refers down her leg in the posterior thigh and into the right posterior calf in a predominately S1 dermatomal distribution. Rebecca's pain is worse with sitting and better with standing. The pain is worse in the morning and worse with transitioning from sit to stand. The pain is 4/10 at best and 9/10 at worst. Rebecca denies any numbness, tingling, or burning sensations in her legs. She does not have left lower back or leg symptoms. She does not note any subjective weakness in her legs. She denies any change in bowel or bladder habits. Other than her pain, Rebecca has always been in very good general medical health.

Over the course of the last several months, Rebecca has been given various pain medications. She has tried Cymbalta, Lyrica, Neurontin, Topamax, Vicodin, Percocet, tramadol, and various NSAIDs. The only medications that she feels really helps her pain are the narcotic medications. Currently, she is taking Percocet 5/325 one tab 3–4 times per day. She says that she hates taking the medication and wants very much to get off of it. She is embarrassed about the medication and feels "like a drug addict." She says that without the pain medication, she cannot function at her job or with her family.

Her husband, who is also an attorney, is very concerned about her and wants her to go on medical disability. He has continually recommended that she "fly somewhere like to the Mayo Clinic or somewhere like that" where they can figure her problem out. Since the second pain management doctor, Rebecca has been to a second spine surgeon who also told her that he could not help her. That spine surgeon suggested that her pain may be coming from her hip. She went to a hip surgeon who told her that her problem was coming from her spine. Her primary care doctor told her that she was depressed and sent her to a psychiatrist. Rebecca says that she does not feel depressed but is "willing to try anything" to get the pain to go away so she went to the psychiatrist.

The psychiatrist is the one who put Rebecca on Cymbalta but that made her feel "very out of it" and she stopped it after only a week. She also went to a clinical psychologist for a month but she did not feel that was helping. Rebecca admits to feeling very frustrated, stressed, and depressed but believes that her psychological symptoms are a result of her pain and not the cause of her pain.

Rebecca has also been to a neurologist. The neurologist performed an EMG/NCS that he told her was normal. The neurologist gave her Topamax but it made her feel very sleepy and so she had to stop it. She went to a rheumatologist who checked "a bunch of lab work including a Lyme test" that was all normal. The rheumatologist said that she could not help and recommended going back to her pain management doctor.

Rebecca has tried two other chiropractors in the last several months. One of them did not help at all. The other chiropractor seemed to be helping at first but then the pain kept returning. Rebecca says that she is at her "wits end" and feels that the pain is ruining her life. Several times during the history taking, Rebecca pauses to dab her teary eyes with tissue paper. She has come to this office, which is a 2 h drive, because a colleague referred her after he had a very positive experience.

Physical Examination

On physical examination, Rebecca is 5′6″ and 115 lb. She has a slim build and exhibits excellent posture. She has a normal gait. She is in obvious discomfort with transition from sit to stand. She has full lumbar flexion but does have pain at about 30–40° of lumbar flexion. She has full lumbar extension but has pain with right lumbar oblique extension but no pain with left lumbar oblique extension.

Rebecca has tenderness over the right lower lumbar paraspinals as well as tenderness to deep palpation of the right quadratus lumborum muscle. Her right sacroiliac joint is tender. Her right piriformis muscle is tender as well although palpation of the piriformis muscle does not reproduce the lower extremity symptoms into the thigh or calf. She has a very tight and tender right iliotibial band.

Rebecca has full range of motion of her hips. She has mild pain with FABER test on the right. Straight leg raise on the right is positive at 40° although the pain that is reproduced is only in the right lower back and buttock and not in the leg, and the severity of the reproducible pain on straight leg is "not terrible." She clearly has tighter knee extensors on the right than the left. She has a negative slump test bilaterally.

Rebecca has 5/5 strength in her lower extremities. She has intact sensation to light touch in her lower extremities. She has brisk and symmetric reflexes in her patella and Achilles reflexes. She has negative Babinski and Hoffman's reflexes bilaterally.

Assessment and Plan

Having heard Rebecca's presentation, what does she likely have and what is the next step that you would take as her treating physician?

Given all of the above, a diagnosis of right L5 and S1 radiculopathy is certainly not unreasonable. A normal electrodiagnostic study argues against a radiculopathy but it does not rule one out. The presence of only a mild right paracentral disc bulge at L5–S1 may easily be an incidental finding and then again is certainly consistent with Rebecca's signs and symptoms. The fact that Rebecca failed to respond to two epidural steroid injections may be because she does not really have a radiculopathy (or radiculitis) or it may be because the radiculopathy is not going to respond well to steroids, or it may be because the injection was performed using an interlaminar approach rather than a transforaminal approach and so perhaps not enough of the medication reached the target location.

Rebecca's physical examination findings are equivocal in that they point to a number of potential pathophysiologic causes without being particularly convincing of any one in particular. The fact that the pain refers along the S1 nerve root dermatome points in the direction of a radiculitis but the disc itself, the facet joint, sacroiliac joint, and piriformis syndrome can all refer pain along the same pattern. Further, the character of the pain is not classic for nerve pain but rather sounds more like a referral pain pattern from a spinal structure such as the disc, facet joint, or sacroiliac joint. At the same time, it is always important to remember that neuropathic pain can take many forms and masquerade as various musculoskeletal or even visceral structures.

What is most notable about Rebecca and what gives Rebecca's presentation the most optimism for an ultimately successful interaction despite her difficult pain history is that Rebecca's pain has not been given the benefit of an evidence-based diagnostic and treatment paradigm. That is to say that the L5 and S1 nerves have been somewhat interrogated with the repeat interlaminar injections and the EMG/NCS, but the other spinal structures do not seem to have even been considered.

All of the above is discussed with Rebecca. It is explained to her that given all she has been through, before trying to empirically manage her pain with chronic medications, it seems most appropriate and optimal to methodically explore the various potential pain generators. Rebecca agrees with all of the above and is excited to learn about her spine and to understand the science behind the potential pain generators and how they can be evaluated. Although she has had two epidurals in the past, it is decided to start with a right L5 and S1 transforaminal epidural steroid injection. This is decided because her history, physical examination, and MRI findings all seem most consistent with this diagnosis and the interlaminar injection may simply have failed to get enough of the medication to desired location.

Follow-Up

Rebecca undergoes the right L5 and S1 transforaminal epidural steroid injection and tolerates the procedure very well. In fact, she has no anesthesia with the injection and experiences very little if any discomfort. This brings up an important point. An epidural that is performed without sedation is not designed to reproduce pain and indeed steps are taken to avoid pain during the procedure. However, anecdotally it may be said that when symptoms are not at all reproduced with a transforaminal epidural steroid injection, many spine specialists who perform injections will take that as a negative predictive factor that the correct pain generator has been found. That is to say that—anecdotally speaking—typically a transforaminal epidural steroid injection, when performed at the correct pain generator, often reproduces at least some of the patient's pain. Nevertheless, Rebecca was given a pain diary following the injection.

Rebecca kept the pain diary for the rest of the day and returned 2 weeks later to discuss her results and experience. She had about a 30 % reduction of pain in the right buttock and leg for about 7 h after the injection. At 8 h the pain had returned to baseline and at 2 weeks she reported feeling "absolutely no better."

Rebecca was disappointed with her lack of response to the epidural steroid injection. She was visibly frustrated to the point of tears. At that point, she was reminded that this was a process and right now, at that moment, she was walking through the limited number of steps necessary to find the pain generator. She was reminded that the injection was not a failure. The injection confirmed that the right L5 and S1 nerve roots were not the pain generators. Learning this had real value as now the next diagnostic steps could be taken.

The next most likely cause of Rebecca's pain, epidemiologically speaking, was her facet joints. As such, the next step that was agreed upon was to inject Rebecca's right L3–L4, L4–L5, and L5–S1 facet joints. Rebecca tolerated the procedure very well. Again, Rebecca kept a pain diary for the rest of the day. On her return visit, Rebecca reported no relief from the lidocaine or the steroid and again she was at her baseline level of pain.

Rebecca again was naturally frustrated. In her case, it was agreed that there were two more potential pain generators—the sacroiliac joint and the piriformis muscle/sciatic nerve—that had a reasonable chance of being responsible for her pain. While her pain pattern was more consistent with piriformis syndrome, the sacroiliac joint was epidemiologically more likely to be responsible for her pain. As such, the next injection that was agreed to be performed was of the right sacroiliac joint.

Rebecca underwent a fluoroscopically guided right sacroiliac joint injection. Rebecca had a moderate amount of pain when the medication was injected into her right sacroiliac joint. When she got up off the table, she started crying in disbelief because for the first time in a really long time, she had 100 % relief of her pain both in her right buttock and also her right leg. Rebecca was reminded to remain skeptical and as aloof as possible to her emotions and just record her pain relief over the rest of the day.

Rebecca returned in 2 weeks with her pain diary. She had experienced 100 % pain relief for two full days before the pain slowly returned to 80 % improvement. At 2 weeks, she was very happy to report that she was still feeling about 80 % better. Rebecca was very nervous that the pain would return and wanted to know the next steps in her treatment.

A pain diary that has the patient feeling 100 % better for more than 8 h is always a little hard to interpret. On the one hand for Rebecca, it certainly seems that the right sacroiliac joint is her pain generator. On the other hand, even a perfect-looking pain diary carries about a 32 % false-positive rate. Knowing that lidocaine does not last 2 days, what accounts for the full pain relief during that time? Did the lidocaine interrupt the pain cycle and that in turn made the pain relief last longer than the chemical action of lidocaine itself? Did the steroids become metabolized extremely quickly and so as the lidocaine was wearing off in a few hours it blended into the action of the steroids to account for the longer pain relief? Is one of the ways that lidocaine blocks the pain a "washout" effect of the inflammatory proteins that may result in longer duration pain relief from the lidocaine alone? Was the pain relief all placebo driven? Could there have been a combination of lidocaine being injected into the correct pain generator and then that combining with the excitement of the pain abating for a few hours and the natural endorphins that might have been released by Rebecca at the realization that her pain may actually be going away and treatable at its source and that she might actually get her life back after so much time with the pain?

The last explanation above seems the most plausible to this author, but there is really a paucity of science to explain the empiric observation that many patients experience longer-lasting pain relief than the actual action of the anesthetic. What may safely be said is that it is reasonable to view with greater skepticism a pain diary response that does not more neatly conform to what is known about the mechanism of action of lidocaine.

Whatever the potential role of placebo in Rebecca's response, she was feeling 80 % better at 2 weeks follow-up. Given her improvement, the various options were discussed with Rebecca but the one that seemed the most appropriate was to send Rebecca back to physical therapy. At first, Rebecca was very reluctant to return to therapy when it had not helped her at all in the past. However, the following three points were made for her.

First, the last time Rebecca went to physical therapy, she went with the diagnosis of lumbosacral radiculopathy. Because of this, it pointed the therapists in the wrong direction and the exercises and passive modalities were focused on the wrong underlying problem.

Second, the major piece that seemed to have been missing from her previous physical therapy program (even if the diagnosis had in fact been a lumbosacral radiculopathy) was a focus on lumbar stabilization exercises.

Third, with 80 % of her pain in her rear-view mirror, Rebecca is now returning to physical therapy to focus more on *learning* a set of exercises tailored for her with an emphasis on lumbar-stabilizing exercises and hip-strengthening exercises. Once she learns the exercises, she may leave therapy and do the exercises on her own. If she learned the exercises quickly, she could leave therapy quickly. Rebecca was concerned about time commitment but she realized after the conversation that she could realistically likely return to physical therapy for only a couple of weeks and then do the exercises on her own.

Rebecca returned 1 year later. She had gone to physical therapy for 3 weeks after the last visit and then felt comfortable with her exercise program. She had been doing her exercises consistently and feeling about 90 % better until 2 months ago when the pain slowly and insidiously began to return. The pain is not as bad as it had been previously, but the pain is about 5/10 on VAS and she says that it has been getting worse every week despite doing her exercises.

On repeat physical examination, Rebecca's exam was virtually identical to her initial examination. It was agreed that the sacroiliac joint injection would be repeated. Again she tolerated the right sacroiliac joint injection well and again she was given a pain diary. She returned for a follow-up evaluation 2 weeks later and reported feeling almost 100 % better. The pain relief started nearly immediately after the injection and persisted at 2 weeks. It was suggested to Rebecca to return to physical therapy to review her home exercises and make sure that her form was perfect and to try adding different exercises as well.

At first, Rebecca did not want to return to physical therapy because she felt that she already knew her exercises. One point that patients sometimes might miss about physical therapy is that sometimes it may be beneficial to return for a few sessions. Sometimes, a patient's exercise form may have lapsed as time goes on. Sometimes the exercises have become stale and the patient needs new ones because (1) the exercises are no longer engaging or challenging and so the patient is at risk of stopping them out of boredom and also because (2) muscles need new exercise patterns to keep them growing and strengthening and becoming more flexible. A physical therapist may be able to add additional exercises to replace older ones that the patient may find more engaging and challenging, delete exercises that might have become too easy, and tighten up form that may have lapsed with time.

Ideally, a patient in Rebecca's situation will have two exercise programs—a longer exercise routine of around 40–60 min and a shorter exercise routine that is made from the longer exercise routine but that the patient may perform 10–15 min a day using different exercises each time to keep the muscles guessing and the patient engaged. Rebecca was reminded of all of these points and she returned to physical therapy as requested.

Rebecca returned 2 months later. She was very disappointed because the pain in the right buttock had returned 3 weeks after her last visit and had been getting steadily worse again. She is very concerned. Nothing in particular seemed to have triggered her pain to come back. She had continued her exercises and not had any major change of routine or trauma, so why had she returned so soon? At 35, Rebecca wants to know if the condition is worsening and if she will need injections every few months for the rest of her life.

With the pain returning so soon, it is difficult to say if the condition is actually worsening, if she was just unlucky this last time, if the condition is changing and now there may be another overlapping pain generator, or if perhaps the diagnosis was never correct in the first place.

At this point, Rebecca has had two diagnostic and therapeutic sacroiliac joint blocks that both seemed to confirm right sacroiliac joint as the diagnosis. However, it must be remembered that both blocks had uncharacteristic pain relief from the lidocaine in that the pain relief lasted much longer than would have been expected from the chemical properties of the anesthetic. Also, the two blocks were separated by a full year.

When dealing with the facet joints, with one diagnostic block there is about a 32 % false-positive rate and that false-positive rate drops to 8 % with two positive diagnostic blocks. It seems reasonable to extrapolate this data and apply it to sacroiliac joints, although it must be remembered that this is an extrapolation. There is no data to report the false-positive rate of two diagnostic blocks separated by a span of more than a year, and so now this is another leap to make in the assumption that the accurate diagnosis for Rebecca has been made.

If the sacroiliac joint were known to be the pain generator, and if the injections were only therapeutically lasting for several weeks, then it would be smart to consider performing a radiofrequency rhizotomy procedure of the sacroiliac joint. However, because the diagnosis remained in some doubt, and because the first injection in combination with the home exercise program lasted over a year, a third sacroiliac joint injection was performed for both diagnostic as well as anticipated therapeutic purposes.

Rebecca returned 9 weeks after the third sacroiliac joint injection. Her experience from the third injection was nearly identical to her experience after the second sacroiliac joint injection. Immediately after the third injection, her pain in the right lower back, buttock, and lower extremity disappeared and she was nearly pain-free. The near-complete pain relief lasted for almost 5 weeks when the pain began to return. Currently, 9 weeks postinjection, her pain level was a 6/10 on VAS. Rebecca's physical examination was largely unchanged.

Given that she had three positive, albeit atypical, responses to lidocaine in the right sacroiliac joint, and given that the therapeutic aspect of the injection was lasting for only a little more than a month at this point despite Rebecca's follow-through with her exercises, it seemed reasonable to perform the radiofrequency rhizotomy of the right sacroiliac joint.

Rebecca asked if she had other options besides "burning the nerves." It was explained to Rebecca that she certainly did have a plethora of other options. She could try acupuncture, chiropractic, more physical therapy, different physical therapies such as aquatic physical therapy, different pain medications, and even another steroid injection. However, in the opinion of her treating physician, proceeding with the radiofrequency rhizotomy seemed to make the most sense at that point for all of the reasons articulated.

Rebecca discussed it with her husband and she decided to have the radiofrequency rhizotomy procedure performed. Using a single probe with three active electrode sites using a preprogrammed sequence that created overlapping spheroid-shaped burn lesions, the radiofrequency rhizotomy of the right sacroiliac joint was performed. Rebecca tolerated the procedure very well.

Rebecca returned for follow-up visit 3 weeks later. She had been sore "for about a week" after the procedure but at follow-up she had 100 % pain relief. She was very happy. She was continuing to do her home exercises and hoped that by doing them, the pain would not return. She understood, though, that on average the nerves may regenerate in 6–18 months and that she may need a repeat procedure.

Fourteen months later, Rebecca did return with a recurrence of the pain. She said that for 12 months she was pain-free. She said that to her disappointment she had not been doing her home exercises. She said that at first after the radiofrequency rhizotomy, she had performed her home exercise routine "maybe 3–4 times per week." However, she said that she had gotten busy at work and slowly stopped doing them after a few months. She understood the importance of performing the home exercises and meant to make them a priority once she was feeling well again.

She was hoping to have the radiofrequency rhizotomy repeated since it had worked so well the first time.

The recurrent pain felt like her previous pain and referred in the same distribution. The pain was 5/10 on VAS. The option of a repeat lidocaine and steroid injection into the right sacroiliac joint was discussed but given how well she tolerated the radiofrequency rhizotomy procedure the first time and given that her symptoms and physical examination were the same as they were prior to the previous radiofrequency rhizotomy, it was agreed that she would undergo the radiofrequency rhizotomy procedure again.

Rebecca tolerated the second radiofrequency rhizotomy of the right sacroiliac joint just as well as the first. Again, at 3 weeks' follow-up, she was pain-free. Rebecca asked to return to physical therapy for a couple of weeks to refresh her memory about her exercises. After that, she would return to her home exercises. She understood that despite the exercises the pain may return but that hopefully it would not either because the nerves were sufficiently burned that they would not regenerate or because she would do a good enough job with her home exercise routine that the biomechanics would improve and the same stresses would not go through the sacroiliac joint in the same way so that the inflammation in the joint would not return.

Chapter 29
Clinical Case #11: Hector

Hector is a 20-year-old football player in his junior year at his state university. Hector developed lower back pain around the beginning of his football season 4 months ago, and the pain has slowly worsened over the course of the season. He remembers the pain starting after one particularly hard practice but he does not remember any particular tackle or injury occurring during that practice. There was no "pop" that precipitated the pain. At first Hector thought that his lower back muscles were "just sore" as they often were, but as the pain persisted and then significantly worsened in the last month, he became worried that something might really be wrong with his lower back.

Hector's lower back pain spreads across his lower back around his L4, L5, and S1 region. The pain does not radiate into the legs. He denies any numbness or tingling in the legs. He denies any subjective weakness in the legs. The pain is constant but is worse when he plays football. The pain is also worse with prolonged standing or prolonged sitting. The pain is worse with rotation of his lumbar spine and he has very bad pain with transitions from sit to stand. Sometimes after a long practice or game the pain becomes so bad that he has a lot of trouble falling asleep at night and then the pain sometimes wakes him up when he does fall asleep.

Hector has not had any imaging studies. He has been to his football team's trainers on multiple occasions and had many massages. Massages help temporarily. Hot packs and ice baths help the pain temporarily. He has been taking 800 mg of ibuprofen three times per day for the last month and he is not sure if that helps or not but he figured it would reduce the inflammation. He has taken some muscle relaxers that a friend of his gave him to try. The muscle relaxers did not help. When asked how he makes it through the game with all of his pain, Hector says that once he starts playing in a game, his adrenaline "takes over" and he doesn't think about the pain. However, after the game he rates his pain in his lower back as 9/10 on VAS. At best, his pain in the last month is 4/10 when taking the 800 mg of ibuprofen and resting.

Hector is very concerned about being able to continue playing football. He has a full football scholarship to his university. He is not thinking of turning professional after college but he says that he needs to keep playing to keep his scholarship. Also,

G. Cooper, *Non-Operative Treatment of the Lumbar Spine*,
DOI 10.1007/978-3-319-21443-6_29

he loves playing football and wants to keep playing for that reason, too. After graduating college, Hector plans on going to graduate school to get his Ph.D. in chemistry. Hector did not want to go to a doctor at first but the lower back pain has been getting worse and affecting his ability to concentrate on his studies and also making it more and more difficult to play football at his top performance level.

Physical Examination

On physical examination, Hector is 6′4″ and 220 lb. He has a muscular frame and walks with a normal gait. With normal transitions from sitting to standing, he is not in obvious discomfort. He has full lumbar flexion. His lumbar extension is restricted and causes a small amount of pain. Bilateral lumbar oblique extension is also restricted and causes significant pain at the end range of his movement.

Hector has minimal tenderness to palpation of his lumbar paraspinals. His sacroiliac joints are not tender. His piriformis muscles are not tender. He has full range of motion of his hips and negative FABER test bilaterally. Straight leg raise is negative bilaterally. Slump test is negative bilaterally. Hector has tight hip flexors but good flexibility in his knee extensors, especially considering his size.

Hector has 5/5 strength in his lower extremities. He has intact sensation to light touch in his lower extremities. He has brisk and symmetric reflexes in his patella and Achilles reflexes. He has negative Babinski and Hoffman's reflexes bilaterally.

Assessment and Plan

Having heard Hector's presentation, what does he likely have and what is the next step that you would take as his treating physician?

Hector has chronic axial lower back pain that may be due to a number of causes. Epidemiologically, an annular tear in one of his discs is the most likely cause. Facet joint pain and sacroiliac joint pain are also likely causes. However, given Hector's age and participation in football, the first thing that has to be ruled out is a pars interarticularis fracture.

Hector's problem was discussed in full with him. Many physicians would initially order X-rays of his lumbar spine, including the important oblique views to help rule out a spondylolysis. However, for Hector, given that his pain is chronic, if the X-rays were positive for a fracture, he would need an MRI or CT to evaluate for staging of the fracture. In the event of a fracture, MRI would be ordered first because it may give all the needed information and does not have the radiation of the CT scan. If the X-rays were negative, Hector would still need an MRI to evaluate his chronic lower back pain anyway. Furthermore, MRI may detect a stress reaction and this of course may be a precursor to a fracture. These findings may be of particular benefit to Hector because it may inform recommendations pertaining to return to play for an athlete in a contact sport. Therefore, given that the MRI would be needed anyway, it was agreed to first obtain an MRI of the lumbosacral spine and avoid the need for the radiation involved with a lumbar spine X-ray series.

Follow-Up

Hector returned with his parents after having his MRI of the lumbosacral spine. Hector's images were reviewed with him and his parents. The MRI revealed mild spondylosis in the L4–5 and L5–S1 facet joints and a small annular tear in the L4–5 and L5–S1 disc. A study in September 2014 revealed that MRI may be *more* sensitive than CT scan for spondylolysis, but there have been many fewer studies on whole about MRI and spondylolysis than CT scans for subtle spondylolysis.

Given the imaging studies, the findings of two annular tears, and the raw epidemiology of discogenic lower back pain in Hector's age group being the cause of chronic lower back pain, the leading presumptive diagnosis for him was discogenic lower back pain. However, because of Hector's high-level participation with football and his desire to continue in football, after a discussion of the relative pros and cons with Hector and his parents, it was agreed that the relative risk of one CT scan was less than the potential to miss a small spondylolysis and return Hector to full contact division I football. A CT scan was thus obtained of Hector's lumbar spine to evaluate specifically for a spondylolysis.

Hector and his parents again returned after the CT. The CT scan was negative for spondylolysis. Hector was naturally relieved about his lack of a stress fracture. Hector was sent to physical therapy to focus on an aggressive program of lumbar stabilization exercises and hip flexor stretching.

At first, Hector and his parents were resistant to the idea of physical therapy. They simply did not believe that someone as strong and muscular as Hector could benefit from physical therapy. In the office, Hector was asked to perform a pelvic tilt. Hector performed this maneuver and then was instructed to hold the pelvic tilt while also performing heeltaps. Immediately, Hector had trouble holding his pelvic tilt while doing this exercise.

Hector was indeed a very strong young man, but the difficulty that he had with the exercise of holding the pelvic tilt and performing heeltaps demonstrated the point that his lumbar stabilizing muscles, while stronger than most, were not as strong or integrated as they could be to protect his spine. He understood this principle and agreed to attend physical therapy. Hector then asked if he could continue with playing football while also going to therapy. Ultimately, Hector agreed to take 2 weeks off of contact football and focus on his physical therapy and then return to contact football afterward and see how he felt.

Hector was also asked to stop taking the ibuprofen 800 mg PO TID as this did not seem to be helping him and had the potential to negatively affect his kidneys and stomach.

Hector went to physical therapy and did extremely well with the therapy as well as the 2 weeks of relative rest. Hector returned to the office in 2 weeks and felt overall 80 % better—although he admitted that he was not sure how much of his pain improvement was from his relative rest from contact football. Hector was cleared to return to full contact football but was asked to listen to how he felt and stop playing if the pain significantly worsened.

Hector returned for follow-up evaluation in 2 more weeks and reported that some of the pain had indeed returned when he went back to football but it was not nearly as bad as before. Overall he estimated that his pain was still about 60 % improved from baseline. Hector was very motivated to continue with his physical therapy for the duration of the season. He asked if it were dangerous for him to play despite the pain.

It was explained to Hector that if his life were devoted to keeping his back healthy, he should stop playing football and focus on his lumbar stabilization exercises. However, if his pain continued to be mild to moderate, if he did not develop neurologic or other symptoms, and if playing football was very important to him, then it was not unreasonable to continue playing for the remainder of the season but that he needed to be honest with himself and his coaches about the intensity of the pain, and he should not try to mask the pain with medications.

Hector decided to continue playing for the rest of the season. He continued with his physical therapy exercises during the off season, and by the end of the academic year, he was glad to report that he had become pain-free. In his senior year, Hector did not have a recurrence of the lower back pain and was able to play his final entire season without event. Hector did not become a professional football player and decided to not become a chemist either. Instead he decided to become a physical therapist.

Hector's pain may have been from discogenic sources, facet joint pain, sacroiliac joint pain, or even another source. Because he did so well with physical therapy and did not have a recurrence of pain, it was never necessary to perform any further diagnostic testing.

Hector asked if he should expect to have problems with his lower back in the future. It was explained to him that once someone has a significant case of lower back pain, if he does nothing else, then he is more likely to have lower back pain again in the future when compared with his age cohort. However, if Hector were to continue with his physical therapy exercises, as he knew he should and planned to do, then he would probably be less likely to have lower back issues in the future as compared with his age cohort.

Index

G. Cooper, *Non-Operative Treatment of the Lumbar Spine*,
DOI 10.1007/978-3-319-21443-6

MIX
Papier aus verantwortungsvollen Quellen
Paper from responsible sources
FSC® C105338

If you have any concerns about our products,
you can contact us on
ProductSafety@springernature.com

In case Publisher is established outside the EU,
the EU authorized representative is:
Springer Nature Customer Service Center GmbH
Europaplatz 3, 69115 Heidelberg, Germany

Printed by Libri Plureos GmbH
in Hamburg, Germany